New Perspectives on

HYPERTENSION

D1827054

New Perspectives on
HYPERTENSION

Adrian J. B. Brady,
Consultant Cardiologist, Glasgow Royal Infirmary, Glasgow, UK

John R. Petrie,
Senior Lecturer, Division of Cardiovascular and Medical Sciences, University of Glasgow
Honorary Consultant Physician, Glasgow Royal Infirmary, Glasgow, UK

ISBN: 1 873413 67 X

©Merit Publishing International

European address:
1st Floor, 35 Winchester Street, Basingstoke, Hants RG21 7EE
Tel/Fax: 01256 841008

Email: merituk@aol.com

American address:
5840 Corporate Way, Suite 200, West Palm Beach, FL 33407
Tel: (561) 697-1116, Fax: (561) 477-4961

Email: meritpi@aol.com

www.meritpublishing.com

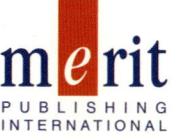

m**e**rit
PUBLISHING
INTERNATIONAL

CONTENTS

AUTHORS

Adrian J.B.Brady, B.Sc (Hons), MD, FRCP(Glasgow), FRCPE, Consultant Cardiologist, Glasgow Royal Infirmary

John R.Petrie, B.Sc (Hons), PhD, FRCP(Glasgow), FRCPE, Senior Lecturer, Division of Cardiovascular Sciences, University of Glasgow and Honorary Consultant Physician, Glasgow Royal Infirmary

Alison Lee, MD, MRCP, Consultant Cardiologist, South Tees Royal Infirmary

Mark Davis, MBChB, General Practitioner, Yorkshire

Neeraj Prasad, MD, FRCP, Consultant Cardiologist, City Hospital, Birmingham

Peter Clarkson, MD, MRCP, Consultant Cardiologist, City Hospital, Birmingham

Stuart Hood, MD, FRCP(Glasgow), Consultant Cardiologist, Royal Alexandra Hospital, Paisley

Jacqueline Taylor, MBChB, FRCP(Glasgow), Consultant Physician, Department of Geriatric Medicine, Glasgow Royal Infirmary

Andrew Clark, MD, FRCP, Senior Lecturer and Honorary Consultant Cardiologist, Hull

Neil Padmanabhan, BSc, MRCP, Registrar in Renal Medicine, Glasgow Royal Infirmary

Mary Joan MacLeod, PhD, Senior Lecturer, Department of Medicine and Therapeutics, Aberdeen University

Ian Greer, MD, FRCOG, Professor of Obstetrics and Gynaecology, University of Glasgow

Neil Chapman, MD, MRCP, Registrar in Cardiology, , St. Mary's Hospital, London

Jamil Mayet, MD, FRCP, Consultant Cardiologist, St. Mary's Hospital, London

Stephen Cleland, BSc, MBChB, PhD, MRCP, Lecturer, in Medicine and Therapeutics, University of Glasgow

Pankaj Sharma, PhD, FRCP Senior Lecturer in Neurology, National Hospital for Nervous Diseases, London

Kennedy R.Lees, MD, FRCP, Professor of Stroke Medicine, University of Glasgow

Henry L. Elliott, MD, FRCP, Senior Lecturer and Honorary Consultant in Medicine and Therapeutics, University of Glasgow

Dean Patterson, MRCP, Registrar, Department of Clinical Pharmacology, University of Dundee

Tom M. MacDonald, MD, FRCP, Professor of Clinical Pharmacology, University of Dundee

FOREWORD

Hypertension is common but, for the primary care practitioners and general physicians who take responsibility for the care of individuals with high blood pressure, its management is not easy. Each year, many books devoted to the topic are published, usually with titles designed to attract the target readership. New Perspectives on Hypertension is unusual in that it really does provide new insights. The authors are young guns from the former British Hypertension Group, most of whom are already authorities in many aspects of the condition, supported in places by established figures in the field. The text is written in language easy to comprehend by the non-specialist, yet it manages to be comprehensive. This slim volume covers in detail the etiology of hypertension, its definition and guidelines for diagnosis. It provides sensible recommendations for investigation and management, and practical advice in a wide range of patient groups.

The importance of considering hypertension as a major but not the only contributor to cardiovascular risk is given prominence. Risk accumulates with the co-existence of risk factors and modern management emphasises global risk assessment and treatment of all reversible risks. Blood pressure reduction is a critical component of risk management strategies.

Many books are obsolescent by the time they are published. This volume is remarkably current with reference to and discussion of important trial results published only in the last few months. New Perspectives on Hypertension is likely to remain a valuable source of pragmatic information for all involved in the management of hypertension for some time.

Gordon T McInnes, MD, FRCP,
Professor of Clinical Pharmacology, Department of Cardiovascular and
Medical Sciences, University of Glasgow.

CHAPTER 1

INTRODUCTION TO HYPERTENSION *Adrian Brady*

Classification of Hypertension
Idiopathic
Essential hypertension (>90% of cases)

Secondary causes
acute and chronic renal disease
Endocrine causes
Other causes
Pregnancy

Definition, Epidemiology and Introduction
Systemic hypertension, hypertension in everyday usage, is a state of sustained high blood pressure. Hypertension is directly associated with stroke, heart disease, renal failure and vascular disease. It is asymptomatic until organ damage is imminent, but easily detectable, and usually can be readily treated. Hypertension results from chronic elevation of the systemic peripheral vascular resistance, a consequence of increased tone within arterioles, the resistance vessels of the systemic circulation. The signals that mediate this chronic constriction are not well understood (see Chapter 2).

In a Western adult population the prevalence of hypertension exceeds 20%. Among some groups, for example black Americans, the prevalence approaches 50% of the middle aged population. Large American surveys have shown about 60% of the entire elderly population to be hypertensive. Hypertension is therefore the commonest chronic condition affecting the adult population in the Western world. The frequency of hypertension is growing in developing nations also.

For most patients who develop hypertension no cause is found; such patients have idiopathic or "essential" hypertension. In fewer than 5% of cases can a clear cause be found with "secondary" hypertension a result. Such patients are often younger, and usually have abnormalities of renal or endocrine function. Hypertension can develop at any stage in life, but most patients with essential hypertension develop the condition in middle age.

Hypertension with onset late in life is increasingly recognized, particularly hypertension with high systolic but relatively normal diastolic values - termed systolic hypertension.

Blood pressure is continuously distributed within populations, skewed towards its upper end. Blood pressure rises with age and levels are therefore defined to categorize individuals as normotensive, borderline or hypertensive. Such levels are defined by the risks of developing organ damage from chronic high blood pressure. These data have been derived from insurance companies' actuarial tables, and from large epidemiological studies.

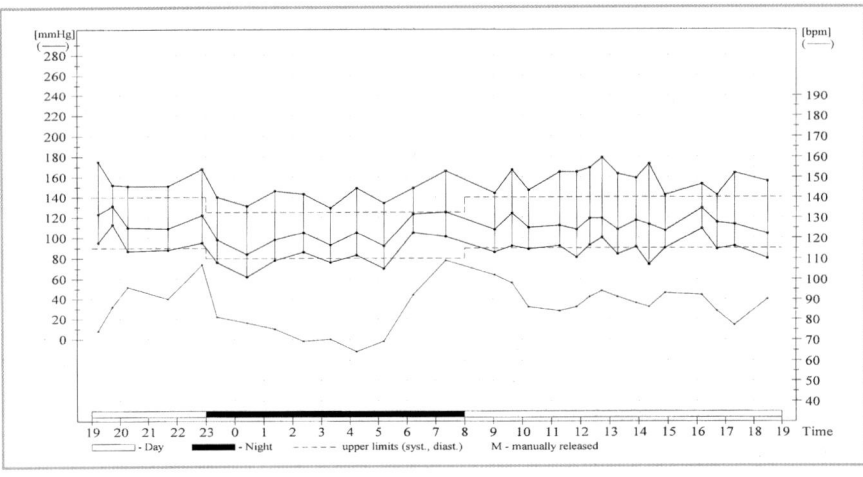

Figure 1. 24-hour ambulatory blood pressure recording of a 54-year-old woman. Note the nocturnal dip, and rise in BP before waking.

Blood pressure varies considerably during the day (see figure 1). Hormonal influences cause an early morning peak. Studies using continuous ambulatory blood pressure monitoring with an indwelling arterial cannula, or intermittent monitoring with a miniaturized recorder and standard cuff, show marked changes with exercise, emotion and stress, and variability at other times with no obvious cause. Blood pressure usually falls at night during sleep. Patients with hypertension usually also show diurnal variation in blood pressure. Some hypertensives do not have a nocturnal fall, and they may be at particular risk of cardiovascular events.

Although this book is about hypertension, the modern strategy for the individual is the appreciation of the total burden of cardiovascular risk for that individual. Age, smoking, cholesterol, a family history of premature cardiovascular disease, and diabetes - as well as hypertension - are the six most important risk factors. Obesity, exercise, diet, socioeconomic factors and comorbid conditions, especially in the elderly, are also crucial. Hypertension is just one risk factor and its importance lies only as one line of attack against the overall cardiovascular risk for an individual. However, among the elderly, blood pressure reduction has greater absolute benefits in preventing stroke and we believe that in this age group especially, hypertension should be sought assiduously and treated to target.

Definition of high blood pressure

Different countries set slightly varying levels at which hypertension is defined. Over recent years more aggressive guidelines have defined high blood pressure at progressively lower absolute levels. The table below condenses current definitions which are internationally acceptable.

Age	normal	borderline	high
<40	<140/85	140-150/85-90	>150/90
41-60	<140/90	140-150/90	>160/90
61-75	<140/90	150-60/90	>160/90
>75	<150/90	160-170/90	>170/90

The reader should note that diabetic patients are likely to live longer and healthier with a low blood pressure. Modern targets aim for a blood pressure < 140/80 mm Hg.. To achieve this usually requires multiple drug therapy.

Natural History

Long term prospective studies in over 420,000 individuals show a direct relationship between elevated blood pressure and increased risk of coronary heart disease and stroke. Even quite modest elevations of 5-10 mm Hg diastolic blood pressure increase the risk of stroke by 40% and heart disease by 30% over ten years. However, these figures relate to the relative risk of these events compared to controls.

The *absolute* risk of such an event was approximately 4% over an eight-year period in the hypertensive individuals. Thus hypertension in the absence of other cardiovascular risk factors or end organ damage is important, but the absolute risk of cardiovascular events is much more serious if there is coexisting diabetes, hypercholesterolemia, continuing smoking habit or evidence of coronary or other atheromatous disease.

Sustained high blood pressure causes accelerated atherosclerosis, with consequent coronary heart disease, heart failure, stroke and renal disease. If untreated, approximately 50% of patients die of heart disease, 33% of stroke, and 10-15% of renal failure.

Complications of hypertension

Cardiac complications:
Left ventricular hypertrophy
Coronary heart disease
Congestive heart failure
Arrhythmias incl. sudden death

Vascular complications:
Stroke
Renal failure
Aortic aneurysm and dissection
Peripheral vascular disease
Hypertensive retinopathy

Causes of Secondary Hypertension

Renal causes - see Chapter 10
acute and chronic renal disease (glomerulonephritis and pyelonephritis)
diabetic nephropathy, analgesic nephropathy)
polycystic kidney disease
renal artery stenosis
polyarteritis nodosa; scleroderma; systemic lupus erythematosis

Endocrine causes - see Chapter 13
Estrogen-containing oral contraceptives
Cushing's syndrome
Conn's syndrome
Congenital adrenal abnormalities (e.g., 11ß hydroxylase deficiency)
Acromegaly
Hypothyroidism
Hyperparathyroidism

Other causes
Coarctation of the aorta - see Chapter 9
Porphyrias
Arteriovenous fistula and patent ductus arteriosus (systolic hypertension)
Raised intracranial pressure (acute HT)
Pregnancy - see Chapter 11

Oral contraceptives
The Estrogen-containing oral contraceptive pill causes a small rise in blood pressure in most women, probably due to renin-angiotensin II – mediated volume expansion. However, only about 5% of users over five years will develop hypertension, about three times more than among non-users. The risk of developing hypertension is greatest in women over 35, the obese and in those who drink excess alcohol. Hypertension in a previous pregnancy also increases the risk of subsequent hypertension with oral contraceptives.

When oral contraceptives are discontinued after hypertension develops, blood pressure falls back to normal over 3-6 months in about half of the women. Among those whose blood pressure remains elevated, it is not known whether the contraceptives precipitated the onset of hypertension that was going to develop later anyway. Low dose estrogens have a lesser hypertensive effect and may be safer. Estrogens as part of hormone replacement therapy (HRT) in postmenopausal women are given at a low dose which does not cause a rise in blood pressure. However, emerging evidence in 2003 suggests that some forms of HRT increase the risk of breast cancer, heart disease, stroke and venous thromboembolism and patterns of HRT use may change sharply in coming years.

Malignant hypertension

Malignant hypertension is still encountered despite improvements in antihypertensive treatment and blood pressure screening. The clinical syndrome is characterized by headache, impaired conscious level, frank neurological signs, nausea and vomiting, acute congestive heart failure, papilledema and oliguria in the presence of a diastolic blood pressure >130-140 mm Hg. The crucial differential diagnosis is from a stroke or subarachnoid hemorrhage with accompanying hypertension, often a feature of acute cerebrovascular events. Hypertensive crisis, with blood pressures typically >200/140 is a medical emergency, requiring hospital admission and frequent monitoring.

However, most patients with severe hypertension can be safely treated with oral agents. Indications for intravenous therapy are encephalopathy, heart failure and myocardial ischemia. The temptation is to administer large doses of potent antihypertensives, but uncontrollable doses of powerful vasodilators may precipitate sudden hypotension with cardiovascular collapse and cerebral infarction. If intravenous therapy is required, for example if there is concomitant heart failure or angina, we believe that intravenous glyceryl trinitrate is the safest therapy. It has a very short half life, is given as an infusion, and is readily controlled. Intravenous labetolol, a combined α and ß-blocker, also has a short half-life and is given as an infusion. It should be avoided in heart failure. If there is any question of evolving stroke, great care must be taken not to produce a rapid fall in blood pressure.

Pathological features of hypertension

Within the heart sustained high blood pressure increases after load, causing hypertrophy and stiffening of the left ventricle. Both systolic contraction and diastolic relaxation are affected. Progressive dilatation ensues, with the development of a low cardiac output and heart failure. The stiff, hypertrophied left ventricle is unable to fill normally in diastole, causing pulmonary congestion. This diastolic failure often precedes ventricular dilatation and can be recognized at echocardiography. The presence of LV hypertrophy indicates a substantially higher risk of cardiac events, both arrhythmias and coronary events, plus stroke, and is an indication for more aggressive antihypertensive therapy.

All antihypertensive drugs are beneficial to some extent against LV hypertrophy by reducing blood pressure, but ARBs and ACE inhibitors are the most effective, by their inhibition of angiotensin II – a potent hypertrophic stimulus.

Hypertension accelerates atherosclerosis, and independently causes vascular damage affecting large and small vessels. Hypertension is thus a major risk factor for coronary heart disease and cerebrovascular disease, particularly in combination with diabetes and cigarette smoking. Transient ischemic attacks and strokes, either due to infarction or hemorrhage, occur more frequently in hypertensives, and are related to the degree of hypertension. Multi-infarct dementia and white matter degeneration (Binswanger's disease) are also associated with hypertension. Involvement of the retinal arterioles is a ready clinical marker of tissue damage (see Table). Grade III changes indicate severe, accelerated hypertension and papilledema malignant hypertension.

Hypertensive renal failure is one of the commonest indications for renal dialysis, particularly in black populations. Prolonged high blood pressure causes intraglomerular hypertension, protein leakage manifest as albuminuria, and a gradual but progressive decline in renal function, as sclerosis of glomeruli develops.

Clinical Features

Essential hypertension is almost always asymptomatic. Symptoms develop when the consequences of hypertension result in organ damage. Therefore early detection requires screening of individuals. Even a casual check is valuable. A single high value is associated with greater cardiovascular risk and should be followed up. Non-specific symptoms for example, headache, dizziness or fainting attacks are often attributed to high blood pressure, but are frequent also in normotensives. If not sought specifically, hypertension passes unrecognized until heart disease, blurring of vision from hemorrhages, stroke or renal failure develops.

Hypertensive retinopathy	
Grade I	↑ tortuosity and narrowing of arteriolar lumen
Grade II	Sclerosis of arteriolar wall (silver wiring) Arteriovenous nipping
Grade III	Rupture of small vessels causing flame-shaped hemorrhages and "cotton wool" exudates
Grade IV	Papilledema

Clinical examination reveals elevated blood pressure. The apical impulse may be displaced if LV hypertrophy and dilatation have occurred. The aortic component of the second heart sound may be loud, and there is sometimes a fourth heart sound. This fourth heart sound disappears with control of blood pressure. Examination of the fundus may reveal hypertensive changes (see table). Grade III changes occur in severe, accelerated hypertension and grade IV changes are diagnostic of malignant hypertension.

Diagnosis of hypertension

Blood pressure varies considerably during the day and depends on many factors including the level of stress of the patient. Blood pressure levels should be determined on at least three occasions over a three month interval. Very high readings, greater than 170/110 mm Hg, should be repeated much earlier and treatment initiated if sustained. If there is evidence of end organ damage, angina or heart failure, treatment should be started without delay. Some individuals find the medical environment particularly stressful, elevating their blood pressure. If "white coat" hypertension is suspected, ambulatory blood pressure monitoring using an automated device is helpful to elucidate the normal blood pressure of the patient away from the stressful environment of the clinic. However, such patients may ultimately develop sustained hypertension and should be followed up.

Measurement of blood pressure

Blood pressure is conventionally measured in the ward or clinic using a mercury column sphygmomanometer. Aneroid equipment fits better in a doctor's bag but is less accurate. With the patient seated comfortably for five minutes, the cuff is fitted snugly around the upper arm, leaving enough room for the stethoscope diaphragm to be placed over the brachial artery. The cuff should be the correct size for the arm, a cuff too small producing a spuriously high reading and a cuff too large a falsely low value. The cuff is inflated above systolic pressure, checked by palpating the radial pulse. With the diaphragm of the stethoscope applied, the pressure is lowered steadily. The level at which the first clear appearance of the tapping sound of systolic blood pressure is noted.

Korotkoff defined five sounds discernible during auscultation of the blood pressure. This first sound (K1) is the earliest. As pressure in the cuff decreases and blood flow increases, the sound becomes first quieter (K II) and then louder (K III). The sound abruptly becomes muffled, defined as stage IV. The sound disappears, and this level of blood pressure is stage V. Blood pressure is conventionally recorded as Stage I/Stage V, e.g. 130/80. This corresponds most closely to intra-arterial recordings. In some high output conditions, for example, aortic regurgitation, Korotkoff phase V cannot be determined, and phase IV is used. This should be indicated in the patient's records, for example, 160/60 (K IV).

Investigations

Baseline investigations should include an ECG to detect LV hypertrophy (see Figure 2). A chest X-ray will detect cardiac dilatation, although this is a rather late finding and we do not routinely order CXRs for individuals with recent onset HT. Serum and urine analysis of renal function and screening for diabetes should be performed. Echocardiography is much more sensitive than ECG or CXR to detect LV hypertrophy, but can be reserved for patients who do not settle on conventional therapy, or patients with more severe hypertension.

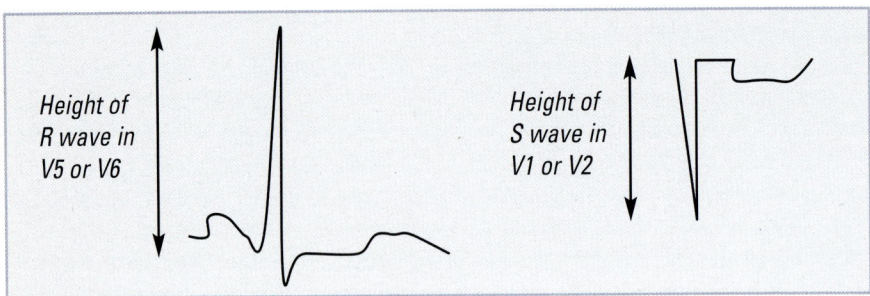

Figure 2. ECG criteria for left ventricular hypertrophy.

ECG diagnosis of LV hypertrophy (LVH)

The hypertrophied left ventricle of LVH generates a larger voltage sometimes detectable on the standard ECG. In adults LVH is suspected when R waves in the leads oriented towards the LV are tall (chest leads V5 and V6, and limb lead aVL), or S waves particularly deep in leads facing the RV (chest leads V1 and V2). The diagram shows that if the sum of the R wave in V5 or V6 and the S wave in V1 or V2 > 37 mm, LVH is present. More severe LVH can cause ST and T wave abnormalities (termed LVH with strain), with ST depression and T inversion. Left axis deviation sometimes occurs as LVH progresses. Figure 3 shows an actual 12 lead ECG from a patient with echocardiographically proven LVH.

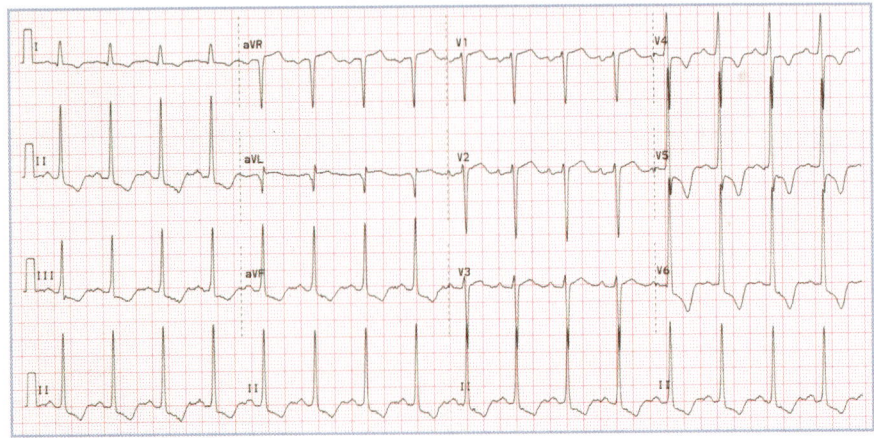

Figure 3. 12 lead electrocardiograph of a patient with hypertension and LVH.

Summary of ECG features of LVH:

- "electrical" LVH ($R_{V5} + S_{V1} > 37$ mm)
- ST depression
- T wave inversion
- left axis deviation

False positive results occur in young thin individuals, particularly men. False negatives are also common, and echocardiography is much more sensitive and specific at detecting LVH.

Investigations for secondary hypertension

Severe hypertension, hypertension which does not respond to conventional therapy, or hypertension in young people should raise the possibility of secondary forms of high blood pressure. Further investigations are then directed towards renal artery stenosis, pheochromocytoma and other rare endocrine conditions. These are discussed more fully in the specific chapters.

Baseline investigations for all patients
ECG
Serum urea, electrolytes and creatinine; cholesterol and glucose should also be measured in most patients
Urinalysis for protein and glucose

Further investigations (see specific chapters)
- Echocardiography - more sensitive test to detect LVH and LV dysfunction
- 24h urine collection for catecholamines
- 24h ambulatory blood pressure monitoring - useful if diagnosis in doubt or suspicion that clinic BP recordings are higher or lower than expected. Figure 1 shows a recording of a patient with rather poorly controlled blood pressure.
- Renal ultrasound or magnetic resonance angiography
- Urine cortisol: creatinine ratio
- serum aldosterone: renin ratio

Hypertension in the elderly(see Chapter 8)

Lowering blood pressure in elderly hypertensives reduces substantially their risk of stroke. They have the most to gain from treatment because stroke is so common in this group.

The prevalence of hypertension among the elderly approaches 50%. Among the elderly, isolated systolic hypertension (ISH) with normal diastolic values has been increasingly recognized, and such patients may account for at least 50% of the elderly hypertensive population. The pathophysiology of ISH is different to the essential hypertension of middle age. Ageing increases the stiffness of the aorta and large conducting vessels. Ejection of blood into the aorta causes a more rapid rise in pressure because of reduced compliance of these large vessels. There is an increase in pulse wave velocity which has an additional effect. Furthermore there is also often a degree of increased peripheral resistance. Because the mechanisms of hypertension are different in ISH, patients may respond differently to anti-hypertensive drugs than patients with essential hypertension. The elderly also have a much greater incidence of side effects. Nevertheless, the incidence of stroke and heart disease is much higher in the elderly, and lowering high blood pressure is of benefit in patients as old as 80-85 years. Beyond this age there are no substantive data from clinical trials. In recent years international guidelines have set progressively lower guidelines on the definition of hypertension in the elderly. Ideally the individual's blood pressure should be below 140/85 mm Hg. Systolic pressure rises with age, and clinical trials have defined values >160 mm Hg as worth treating. Others consider this too aggressive. We believe that a sustained blood pressure >160/90 mm Hg merits therapy, since the reduction in risk of stroke is substantial. Levels of 140-160/95-100 mm Hg should be observed, unless there is end organ damage.

Principles of antihypertensive treatment
The purpose of treating high blood pressure is to prevent the complications of sustained hypertension. Large gains have been made in the reduction in the risk of stroke, with about a 40% reduction in risk. The effect on coronary heart disease has been less impressive, with a risk reduction of about 20%. Hypertension is readily identifiable and treatable, unlike other cardiovascular risk factors, for example a positive family history, and we believe that such an important therapeutic possibility should always be pursued.

The "J" shaped curve
Much harm has been done by physicians obsessed by the possibility of lowering blood pressure too much. Undertreatment of hypertension exposes the patient to an ongoing risk of stroke and heart disease. The belief in a J shaped curve, where a low blood pressure puts the patient at higher risk is not based on any robust evidence. The new trials with aggressive blood pressure lowering show the safety and large benefit of lower achieved pressures. We should not lower diastolic blood pressure to levels < 55 mm Hg, but in practice this is rarely a problem. Over exuberant blood pressure lowering will be announced by postural dizziness. In real life, lowering systolic blood pressure by 15-20 mm Hg will reduce stroke risk by 50%. This is usually readily achievable.

Why does lowering BP in a hypertensive not reduce risk to that of a normotensive person?
This is an unanswered question. Most likely, because the achieved blood pressures in major clinical trials do not ever quite reach normal. Also, when well treated hypertensives are tested on a treadmill, their exercise BP is often still higher than a normotensive individual. How to remedy this without causing postural hypotension is by no means easy. Furthermore, there is no trial in hypertension at the time of writing in 2003 where cholesterol has been treated correctly.

Our belief is that there may be a long term synergism between high blood pressure and high cholesterol where the presence of both is much worse than either alone. In real practice I am as aggressive with cholesterol as with blood pressure. Lowering both substantially will make our patients live longer.

General Measures of antihypertensive therapy

Patients with mild hypertension should be encouraged to adopt a healthy lifestyle if possible. Obesity should be treated, since weight loss is accompanied by a reduction in blood pressure approximating 1 mm Hg for 1 kg. Exercise should be pursued actively. Most importantly, stopping smoking is the most beneficial action. Smoking is an even greater risk factor than hypertension in cardiovascular disease and this should be made clear to the patient. Alcohol intake should be moderated and hyperlipidemia addressed. Women receiving the oral contraceptive pill should switch to a different method of contraception. Salt reduction may be of value in some patients.(see also ACE inhibitors below) Special diets have been proposed but have not proven widely successful. Nevertheless, careful attention to lifestyle produces modest falls in blood pressure and so should be reinforced.

Specific antihypertensive therapy

Most patients, other than previously obese slimmers, will require drug therapy. Treatment is usually lifelong - hypertension usually returns inexorably if antihypertensive therapy is withdrawn. While recent large trials in hypertension have shown important gains against stroke and myocardial infarction, risks have not been reduced to that of the normotensive population. Modern therapy is now aimed at a greater reduction in blood pressure to achieve normal levels, in the hope that the risks of hypertension will be reduced further.

Tailored therapy in Hypertension

Patient group	Diuretic	Beta blocker	calcium antagonist	ACE inhibitor	All blocker (ARB)
No other risk factors	+	+	+/-	+/-	+/-
Hyperlipidemia	-	+/-	+	+	+
Angina pectoris	+/-	++	++	+	+/-
Previous MI	+/-	++	+	++	+/-
Heart failure	++	+*	+/-	++	++
Diabetes	+	+	+	++	++
Renal disease	+	+	+	++**	++**
LV hypertrophy	+	+	+	++	++

* May be valuable in carefully selected cases ** Contraindicated in some cases

There are six main groups of drugs in widespread use, five of which are supported by evidence: thiazide diuretics, ß-blockers, calcium antagonists, ACE inhibitors and angiotensin receptor blockers (ARBs). Alpha blockers are still favored by some physicians, although without long term supportive evidence (see table). Most of the available evidence from older clinical trials examined thiazides and ß-blockers.

There is recent evidence for calcium antagonists, exciting new evidence for ACE inhibitors and especially angiotensin receptor blockers. Calcium antagonists, ACE inhibitors and angiotensin receptor blockers are newer and better tolerated, but are more expensive. Since patients remain on antihypertensive therapy for many years, the cost implications are considerable. Some patients are treated successfully and cheaply with a thiazide or ß-blocker, but many will experience disagreeable side effects and we believe that tailored therapy for these individuals is the most appropriate strategy.

The goal of antihypertensive therapy is to lower blood pressure to normal without side effects. Older textbooks suggest that 75% of hypertensives are successfully treated with a single agent. This is now known to be not true. To achieve modern target blood pressures, 50% of patients will require more than one drug, and the challenge is to find the correct balance for the individual. High doses of single agents cause side effects, and the combination of lower doses of two agents can often avoid this.

Our view is that there is very rarely any indication to use other than once-daily drugs, except for methyl dopa in pregnancy.

Thiazide Diuretics
Thiazide diuretics have been available for over 30 years and remain first line therapy for many patients. They increase sodium excretion by the kidney. Peripheral resistance falls due to a reduction in Ca^{2+} within vascular smooth muscle. High doses cause a greater diuresis and more side effects but no greater antihypertensive effect. Thiazides, especially in higher dose, have a number of unwelcome metabolic effects. Serum potassium falls by 0.5-1 mmol/l, which may precipitate arrhythmias in susceptible patients or patients receiving digoxin. Cholesterol and uric acid may rise slightly with thiazide therapy. Insulin resistance may be increased. Impotence is common in men and can lead to poor compliance. Thus while thiazides have been the backbone of hypertension for many years, their side effect profile has been emphasised as other classes of drugs have become available. Nevertheless, they are useful alone or with vasodilators which cause fluid retention.

Low dose thiazides are well tolerated in the elderly and the diuretic effect can again be useful. Indapamide is a newer agent with a better metabolic profile and fewer side effects, and appears to be better tolerated than older thiazides. The huge ALLHAT study of 2002 showed that thiazide diuretics are still a vital and important class of drugs for hypertension, and remain as first line therapy for many patients.

Beta-adrenergic blockers

ß-blockers have been standard therapy for 20 years. They reduce cardiac output by 15-20% by reducing heart rate and contractility, reduce renin release and inhibit adrenergic neuronal discharge in the CNS. They are particularly useful if there is coexisting myocardial ischemia or if stress is a factor. They work well with diuretics and vasodilators, both of which may increase renin secretion and provoke reflex tachycardia. Newer ß1 - specific drugs are preferred, but must still be avoided in patients with airways disease, peripheral vascular disease and diabetes. ß-blockers reduce contractility, can precipitate heart failure and usually should be avoided in patients with acute LV dysfunction. Emerging research, however, suggests a growing role in selected patients with LV impairment (see treatment of Hypertension and Heart Failure). Fatigue is the most common side effect of ß-blockers, caused by the reduced cardiac output and by central neurological effects. ß-blockers are less effective than thiazides, calcium channel blockers and ARBs in systolic hypertension.

Vasodilator Agents

Practically all other antihypertensive drugs act by causing vasodilatation of vascular smooth muscle. Most act directly on arterioles. Nitrates and alpha-blockers are potent venodilators also, an effect used in the treatment of heart failure. Some drugs act on the central nervous system to affect central regulation of blood pressure.

Calcium antagonists

These are the most widely prescribed antihypertensives in the USA. Felodipine, once daily preparations of nifedipine, amlodipine and diltiazem have substantial evidence to support their use. They act on L-type calcium channels in smooth muscle to inhibit calcium entry. Nifedipine, verapamil and diltiazem are the three prototypes. Within the heart cardiac myocytes and conducting tissue also express L-type calcium channels, and the specificity of drugs varies with regard to the affinity for myocardial, conducting and peripheral vascular calcium channels.

Verapamil in particular affects conducting tissue, reducing conduction velocity and reducing the intrinsic pacemaker rate. This property is used in the treatment of some arrhythmias and angina. Diltiazem also has an effect reducing ventricular rate. Other calcium antagonists have a neutral effect on heart rate, or may cause reflex tachycardia from vasodilatation.

Because they reduce calcium entry into cardiac myocytes calcium antagonists can be negatively inotropic. Patients with heart failure may develop worsening symptoms particularly with verapamil and diltiazem, and most calcium channel blockers can exacerbate the symptoms of heart failure. Amlodipine may be safer than other agents in such patients. All calcium antagonists, like all vasodilators, can cause peripheral edema in a minority.

Calcium channel blockers (and diuretics) are effective in Afro-Caribbean patients. ß-blockers and ACE inhibitors are less effective in this patient group because these patients have lower renin levels. Calcium antagonists are powerful drugs that are best used in sustained release or once daily formulations. Short acting preparations can cause a precipitous fall in blood pressure and are contraindicated in hypertension. Indeed, in 1995 an outcry occurred when a meta-analysis of uncontrolled or poorly performed clinical trials was published, suggesting possible risks of calcium channel blockers in post MI patients. Subsequent analysis of these, together with newer, larger, well conducted trials have shown safety and important benefit from long acting preparations of calcium antagonists, including once daily nifedipine, amlodipine, isradipine, nitrendipine and felodipine in hypertensive patients.

ACE Inhibitors

The renin-angiotensin system can be blocked in three sites, as shown in Figure 4. ACE converts inactive angiotensin I to the active octapeptide angiotensin II. The ACE enzyme has other actions, and catalyses the metabolism of circulating vasodilator kinins. Indeed, ACE inhibitors were first discovered as potentiators of bradykinin, and the realization that the synthesis of angiotensin II could be inhibited came later. Captopril was the first to be developed, followed by enalapril and many newer agents. They all lower blood pressure and are effective at reversing left ventricular hypertrophy, although ARBs maybe better still. They can have a powerful first dose effect in patients

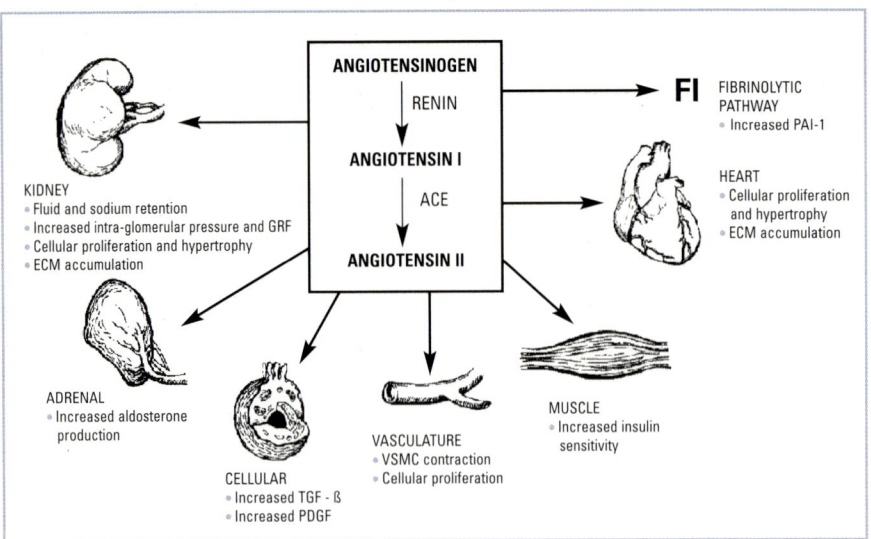

Figure 4. The renin angiotensin system. Conversion of angiotensin I to angiotensin II is inhibited by ACE inhibitors which inactivate the ACE enzyme. Angiotensin II has multiple effects on target organs.

receiving diuretics, and so the starting dose is small. Reducing angiotensin II levels within the kidney reduces efferent arteriolar tone and consequently intraglomerular pressure. ACE inhibitors therefore preserve renal function in diabetics to an important degree. However, by the same mechanism they reduce renal perfusion substantially in renal artery stenosis and should be avoided in this condition.

The main side effect of ACE inhibitors is a dry cough, related to the increased level of circulating bradykinin. Angioneurotic edema rarely occurs; rashes and alteration in taste occasionally occur. Reducing salt intake to foods can have a particular benefit with ACE inhibitor therapy.

Angiotensin II receptor blockers (ARBs)

These drugs, which block the action of angiotensin II at its receptor are now emerging as a leading therapy in hypertension. New long term data show that losartan, the first to be released, had impressive advantages over ß-blocker based therapy in patients with hypertension and LVH. Candesartan also has recently been shown to be of benefit in elderly hypertensives. Angiotensin II receptor blockers are effective and very well tolerated. They do not affect bradykinin and do not cause cough.

As well as for hypertension, these drugs may become valuable in patients with heart failure who can not tolerate ACE inhibitors and they may be especially beneficial in diabetics. They still carry the same risk as ACE inhibitors in patients with renal artery stenosis. While inhibition of renin release has been achieved experimentally, no clinically useful renin inhibitors have been developed to date.

Alpha-adrenergic blockers

These drugs act on post synaptic α_1 receptors causing arteriolar and venous dilatation. They all can cause first dose hypotension. Side effects of dizziness, dry mouth and impotence may be a problem, but the drugs are safe in renal failure and diabetes. Lipids are not adversely affected. They may be useful as second or third line therapy in elderly men where α_1 blockade also relieves muscular tension within the prostate. There is no evidence yet, however, from long term trials of the safety and reduction in stroke and coronary events from these drugs. Indeed, evidence from the large ALLHAT study of 2002 suggested that alpha blockers may be inadvisable as first line therapy.

Other antihypertensive drugs

Directly acting vasodilators - Hydralazine is occasionally used in renal patients, but can cause a SLE-like syndrome. Minoxidil, a potassium channel opener, is very powerful but causes hypertrichosis (hair growth), and is limited to the most refractory renal cases.

Some older drugs act centrally within the central nervous system. Methyldopa, an alpha receptor agonist which reduces CNS sympathetic outflow, is still used widely for hypertension in pregnancy. Longer term use is rare nowadays, because of autoimmune side effects. Moxonidine is a new antihypertensive that acts on alpha1 adrenergic receptors within the central nervous system to reduce sympathetic tone. It appears to be effective and well tolerated, with fewer side effects than older centrally acting drugs. Long term data are not yet available, although it may not be advisable if the patient has heart failure.

Newer drugs are emerging that block the angiotensin system and also prevent breakdown of the endogenous peptide, atrial natriuretic peptide (ANP). ANP promotes Na^+ excretion from the kidney and circulating levels of ANP are increased when ANP breakdown is blocked. This augments Na^+ excretion and provides additional BP lowering effect. Clinical trials are underway, although emerging data are lukewarm rather than exciting.

Endothelin, an endogenous endothelium-derived vasoconstrictor peptide like angiotensin II but more potent and with a longer half life, is a tempting target for antihypertensive drugs but antagonists are still in development.

Antihypertensive drugs in common use

Thiazide diuretics:
bendrofluazide 2.5 mg daily
chlorthalidone 12.5-25 mg daily
hydrochlorothiazide 25-50 mg (sometimes with a potassium-sparing diuretic)
indapamide 1.5-2.5 mg daily

ß-blockers:
atenolol 25-100 mg daily
metoprolol 50-200 mg once-twice daily
propranolol (slow release) 80-240 mg daily
bisoprolol 2.5-10 mg daily

Calcium antagonists:
nifedipine (slow release) 20 mg once daily - 90 mg once daily
amlodipine 5-10 mg daily
felodipine 5-10 mg daily
verapamil (slow release) 120-240 mg daily
diltiazem (slow release) 120-300 mg daily

ACE inhibitors:
captopril 12.5-50 mg three times daily
enalapril 5-40 mg daily
lisinopril 5-40 mg daily
perindopril 2-8 mg daily
ramipril 5-10 mg daily

Angiotensin II receptor blockers (ARBs):
losartan 50-100 mg/daily
valsartan 80-160 mg/daily
candesartan 4-16 mg/day
irbesartan 150-300 mg/day

Alpha-blockers:
doxazosin (slow release) 4-8 mg daily

Six common groups of antihypertensive drugs
thiazide diuretics
beta adrenergic blockers
calcium antagonists
angiotensin converting enzyme inhibitors
angiotensin II receptor blockers
alpha adrenergic blockers

other directly acting peripheral vasodilators - nitrates, hydralazine, minoxidil
centrally acting vasodilators - methyldopa, moxonidine
other drugs - phenoxybenzamine, phentolamine

Summary box 1
Hypertension is the commonest chronic medical condition in the developed world
Hypertension is rare in children; it becomes increasingly common throughout life
>60% of elderly people are hypertensive
The etiology of essential HT is not established
Sustained HT can lead to stroke, heart disease, aortic aneurysm and renal failure

Summary box 2
Secondary hypertension is most commonly due to chronic renal disease
Adrenal and other endocrine causes of HT are rare
<10% of pregnant women develop transient HT;
Eclampsia is rare but is a true emergency
Estrogen containing OCP causes HT in 5% of users after 5 years' therapy
Postmenopausal estrogen HRT may increase cardiovascular and breast
cancer risk

Summary box 3

Tests in essential HT may be often normal

Presence of LVH, renal or fundal damage identifies patients at higher risk

Ageing causes sclerosis (stiffening) of vessels with a consequent rise in systolic pressure

Isolated systolic HT is common in the elderly

Treatment of HT in the elderly has a major and substantial effect reducing stroke

Summary box 4

Non-pharmacological therapy should be tried, but drugs are usually needed

Long term compliance is crucial

HT usually returns if therapy is stopped

Many different classes of drugs are available

Thiazides and ß-blockers are cheap and effective but have many side effects

Newer drugs are better tolerated, but are more expensive

To achieve normal pressure may require a combination of two or more drugs in up to 50% of patients

Summary box 5

Diabetes and HT are a powerful cause of vascular disease

Diabetics with HT should aim for a normal BP

Control of hypertension is at least as important as tight blood glucose control

ARBs are 1st line therapy in hypertensive diabetics with LVH

Summary box 6

HT is very common in the elderly

Treatment will reduce stroke and heart disease

Thiazides, some calcium channel blockers and angiotensin II receptor blockers are proven to be effective in isolated systolic hypertension

CHAPTER 2

ETIOLOGY AND NATURAL HISTORY OF HYPERTENSION *John Petrie*

High BP is not so much a disease as a condition, which predisposes to complications, particularly stroke and myocardial infarction (MI). People are understandably perplexed when they go to their doctor with a headache and are told they should take a tablet (which may make them feel worse) for the rest of their days. It is tempting for doctors and nurses to think of hypertension as a disease, which is either present or absent (like epilepsy or asthma) but this can be misleading.

A good analogy is with height. Just as some people are tall and others short, some have high and others low BP. Tall people have a higher risk of banging their heads when walking through a low doorway, but there is no exact height at which being tall becomes dangerous. The overall risk depends on a number of other factors. A small minority of tall people have a specific endocrine disease state (gigantism) but most are simply at the upper end of the normal height distribution (adult height being determined by the interaction of a host of genetic and environmental factors). While these statements are absurdly obvious, the same concepts are harder to grasp when applied to a variable - blood pressure - which is detected only by auscultation during release of an inflated cuff around the upper arm.

Chronic elevation of systemic peripheral vascular resistance as a consequence of increased tone within arterioles (the "resistance" vessels of the systemic circulation) is a final common pathway in hypertension. Long term prospective studies show a direct relationship between elevated BP and increased risk of stroke and MI. A person with a systolic BP 170 mmHg has twice the cardiovascular risk of a person with systolic BP 120 mmHg. Elevations of 5-10 mm Hg diastolic BP increase the risk of stroke by 40% and heart disease by 30% over ten years. As MI is a more common condition, the greatest burden of hypertension is reflected in coronary artery disease in large numbers of people with modest elevations of blood pressure. Sustained high BP causes accelerated atherosclerosis with consequent coronary heart disease, heart failure, stroke and renal disease. If untreated, approximately 50% of patients die of heart disease, 33% of stroke, and 10-15% of renal failure.

Mechanisms of blood pressure control

A complex set of neural and hormonal systems interact with the mechanical properties of the vasculature to regulate BP according to physiological requirements:

The *sympathetic nervous system* causes peripheral vasoconstriction via α1-receptors, vasodilation via ß2- receptors, and increased heart rate (and cardiac output) via ß1-receptors - the balance is set by a number of reflexes and by higher centers.

Renal sodium handling central to cardiovascular control, is under the influence of the renin-angiotensin-aldosterone hormone system (effected by the pressor hormone angiotensin II and the salt-retaining mineralocorticoid hormone aldosterone), the sympathetic nervous system, and hormones (natriuretic peptides) released by the chambers of the heart.

Catecholamines (adrenaline, noradrenaline) are released into the bloodstream from the adrenal glands and from nerve terminals: these act on the above-mentioned receptors of the sympathetic nervous system.

Endothelial (lining) cells of all blood vessels produce both vasoconstrictor (endothelin, angiotensin II) and vasodilator substances (nitric oxide, prostacyclin, "endothelium-derived hyperpolarizing factor") which regulate local vascular tone. The interaction over time of these control systems is that the average BP of individuals in a population follows a normal frequency distribution.

Those individuals defined as having hypertension (at any point in time) are those whose sustained BP is higher than a value above which (current) evidence suggests that the risks of (current) methods of treatment are outweighed by the benefits – in terms of decreased risk of stroke and/or MI - as demonstrated by high quality randomized controlled trials.

- **Secondary hypertension**
  This occurs in around 5% of cases of hypertension i.e. high BP results from a specific known disorder (Table 1). These conditions are dealt with in chapters 11 (renal) and 13 (endocrine).

- **Essential hypertension**
  When a specific disorder causing elevated peripheral vascular resistance cannot be identified, the term "essential" hypertension is used. Given the complex interacting systems responsible for the physiological regulation of BP, it is likely that this is a heterogeneous state with different pathophysiological mechanisms predominating in different individuals. At present, antihypertensive agents which

work via a variety of mechanisms are prescribed without consideration of the putative cause of high BP in the individual patient: this approach is demonstrably effective if not optimal. Better understanding of the mechanisms by which common variations at genetic loci interact with particular environmental influences to produce high BP via common intermediate phenotypes may lead to more specific forms of antihypertensive therapy for individual patients in the future - this may, in turn, result in more effective prevention of cardiovascular complications.

A number of hypotheses have been proposed for common mechanisms in essential hypertension on the basis of observed differences between hypertensive and normotensive subjects. In most studies, there is considerable overlap between cases and controls. This may reflect in part the heterogeneity of the condition and in part the philosophical problem of grouping patients with different severity (and even causes) of high BP together as a single group. In many cases of hypertension, several of the mechanisms suggested below may be relevant.

Genetic factors: BP (whether high or low) can "track" from parents to offspring. Twins show a high concordance of BP levels, suggesting that inherited factors account for about 25% of the variability in BP. Essential hypertension itself often runs in families. It is conceivable that pressures on survival in past millenia resulted in evolutionary adaptation to environmental factors which are no longer relevant, leading to a predisposition to high BP (by one or more mechanisms).

Birth weight: Epidemiological research has linked low birth weight and subsequent hypertension in adulthood: indeed, it has been suggested that the shared intra-uterine environment of twins may account for some of the variability in BP previously attributed to genetic factors. If the relationship is causal, the underlying physiological mechanisms remain unclear. It is possible that subtle abnormalities of development in the kidneys and/or small blood vessels results in increased sensitivity to hypertensive stimuli in later life. Alternatively, it has been suggested that the association is explained by decreased placental levels of the "shuttle" enzyme (11ß-hydroxy steroid dehydrogenase) which protects the fetus from the mineralocorticoid action of cortisol.

Salt: Decreased dietary salt lowers BP in most individuals, but some individuals who have a more marked drop in BP during salt restriction have been classified as "salt-sensitive." These individuals do not appear to have an overactive renin-angiotensin system but may instead have a genetic variation which causes impaired renal sodium handling (one candidate is a locus encoding a protein known as a-adducin).

Obesity is associated with hypertension, and BP falls when overweight people with hypertension diet successfully. These individuals have high circulating insulin levels and there is evidence that underlying resistance to insulin action may be directly related to increased peripheral vascular resistance.

Insulin resistance is not only present in obese patients and may contribute to high BP even in lean subjects, possibly via a failure of insulin's vasodilator action to balance increased sympathetic nervous system activation resulting from compensatory hyperinsulinemia. Insulin resistance is thought to account for the increased prevalence of hyperlipidemia and diabetes in people with hypertension.

Endothelial dysfunction: Impaired capacity of these vascular "lining" cells (see above) to synthesis NO is present in some cases of hypertension; decreased or increased production of other endothelial factors may be also be important.

Sympathetic nervous system: Early studies suggested that primary over activity of this system might be the cause of high BP; however, this may have been an artefact of using control subjects who were more at ease in the environment in which they were studied (hospital staff).

Emotional stress: may elevate BP in the short term, but is not thought to be the cause of essential hypertension. It is not directly correlated with the "white coat" phenomenon (see Chapter 1). Migration from a relaxed rural environment to the city is associated with a rise in BP but this may be explained by other factors such as changes in diet (salt), exercise, and alcohol intake. Hypertension, and indeed the "physiological" rise in BP with age, are rarely observed in nuns in "closed" orders.

Alcohol: Small amounts may be good for the cardiovascular system but larger amounts taken chronically elevate BP, partly by an increase in sympathetic activity.

● Mechanical properties of the vasculature
Essential hypertension may result from an individual's abnormal response to repeated transient hypertensive influences. In some apparently predisposed individuals, changes in blood vessel structure (hypertrophy) ensue; as hypertrophied vessels are more sensitive to vasoconstrictor substances, a positive feedback system develops. Thus, patients with secondary hypertension in whom the cause is removed after a period of uncontrolled hypertension often develop residual essential hypertension as a result of "structural changes."

Similarly, rat pups exposed to infusions of pressor agents in infancy remain hypertensive lifelong. When local tissue ischemia occurs in the renal vasculature as a result of increased arteriolar tone or hypertrophy, compensatory release of angiotensin II exacerbates the situation.

Many growth factors have been suggested as potentially important mediators of vascular hypertrophy. Secondary hypertension from renal, endocrine or metabolic disease is characterized by well-defined growth promoters, including angiotensin II, growth hormone and catecholamines. How much these contribute to the development and maintenance of the vascular changes in essential hypertension is not firmly established, and is the subject of considerable research.

Hypertensive crises

Awareness of the state of "malignant" or "accelerated" phase hypertension often causes concern in health professionals encountering patients with high diastolic blood pressure readings (>120 mmHg). However, probably because of earlier detection and therapy, few patients now have true accelerated phase hypertension. These patients usually have very high pressures (e.g. > 140 mmHg diastolic), very abrupt rises in pressure, and Grade III or IV retinopathy (Chapter 3); they may have encephalopathy or pulmonary edema.

As the endothelial cell layer of the vessel wall is breached by plasma constituents, there is swelling, reduced lumen diameter and widespread microinfarction (particularly in the retina and kidneys). These patients should no longer be given sublingual or oral short-acting nifedipine capsules as these may cause dangerous precipitous drops in BP.

As cases are rare, there are few relevant trials, but we have used (initially low dose) oral ß-blockers and ACE inhibitors successfully (although the possibility of underlying renal artery stenosis should be considered). If patients are unable to swallow tablets, careful parenteral treatment with nitrates or nitroprusside may be useful initially.

If stroke has developed, extreme caution should be exercised prior to giving any BP lowering therapy as stroke itself can result in adaptive compensatory increases in blood pressure (cerebral autoregulation) which may be disrupted by therapy - in individual cases it may be difficult to decide what is "cause" and what is "effect."

Causes of hypertension	Pathophysiology	Percentage of cases	Chapter
Primary Essential	Unknown	90%	2,4
Secondary Renal disorders: - glomerulonephritis - diabetic nephropathy - pyelonephritis - polycystic kidney disease - connective tissue disorders	Decreased sodium excretion, increased renin secretion		11
Renovascular disease - atheromatous - fibromuscular hyperplasia	Excessive renin secretion	5%	11
Primary hyperaldosteronism Dexamethasone-suppressible hyperaldosteronism	Excessive adrenal aldosterone sectretion (adenoma, hyperplasia)	< 1%	13
Pheochromocytoma	Excessive adrenal catecholamine secretion		13
Coarctation of the aorta	Associated with Turner's Syndrome - also sporadic		13
Cushing's syndrome	Excessive adrenal cortisol production		13
Drugs - Steroids - Combined oral contraceptive	Mineralocorticoid action		13
Miscellaneous endocrine: - Primary hyperparathyroidism - Thyroid disease - Acromegaly			12
Pregnancy			

Key points

- Hypertension is a condition of elevated systemic peripheral vascular resistance

- Sustained high BP causes atherosclerosis with consequent coronary heart disease, heart failure, stroke and renal disease.

- In 95% of cases ("essential hypertension") the exact cause is not currently identified.

- An inherited predisposition to one of a range of environmental factors sets up a positive feedback loop via hypertrophy of small blood vessels

CHAPTER 3

MANAGEMENT OF HYPERTENSION IN THE "UNCOMPLICATED" PATIENT *John Petrie and Adrian Brady*

Although adults should have their BP checked every five years until the age of 80 years, hypertension is often detected during a consultation about an unrelated complaint. If the diagnosis is subsequently established, blood pressure lowering treatment is known to reduce risk of mortality from stroke and myocardial infarction (MI). However, at present many people are unaware of their condition or consider it an unimportant consequence of "stress." In addition, many who do start on treatment do not reach target BP levels - or just stop treatment.

It is often said that the "rule of halves" still applies i.e. at community level at least a third of cases of hypertension are undiagnosed, a third of those diagnosed are not on treatment, and a third of those on treatment are poorly controlled. Although this is a useful rule of thumb, a recent re-analysis of the NHANES cohort in the US has revealed that many patients with untreated or inadequately controlled hypertension are in fact regularly attending (and having BP checked by) a physician. Systolic blood pressure is a better predictor of cardiovascular risk than diastolic blood pressure. This is particularly true in the elderly, who are by far the largest group of individuals with hypertension. Pulse pressure is also a good predictor of events, but is not independent of systolic pressure. Young patients and hypertensive pregnant women may have high diastolic pressure with less marked systolic hypertension.

As hypertension is an asymptomatic condition, finding cases and monitoring compliance/ response to therapy requires excellent local systems of communication amongst patients, family doctors, and hospital specialists – "managed clinical networks." The situation is further complicated by the observation that reducing BP with current drugs does not lower risk of MI to that associated with the level of BP achieved. This may be due to poor attention to other risk factors, principally cholesterol. Careful study of the major hypertension trials shows poor attention to cholesterol in every trial published up to November 2002.

An individual patient who has high BP may or may not be referred for specialist assessment according to local arrangements. Unfortunately, few people are sufficiently well-informed to know if their BP is optimally managed. If it "settles" on the second or third reading, they may not re-attend. As both thresholds and targets for BP treatment are defined on the basis of benefit and risk (and are continuously refined on the basis of emerging data), it is difficult for a general practitioner – with multiple other demands on time - to apply the latest recommendations to their changing population. Liaison with a local specialist is highly desirable and not just for "complicated" cases: mild hypertension and isolated systolic hypertension in the elderly are under-recognized in non-specialist settings.

A number of different guidelines support the process of care e.g. the third working party of the British Hypertension Society (BHS, 1999). As a rule, recent recommendations are based less on the level of BP and more on the level of absolute cardiovascular risk. This is because larger benefits of therapy are seen in those at higher risk. For example, if antihypertensive treatment reduces relative risk of a cardiovascular event by 20%, then a patient who has a baseline absolute ten-year risk of 40% will have an 8% reduction in absolute risk. A patient who starts with a risk level of 10% will only have a 2% reduction i.e. quarter of the benefit. Therefore, 12 patients like our first patient (and 50 patients like our second patient) would need to be treated for 10 years to prevent one event. In fact, trials to-date suggest that it is necessary to treat 70 young low-risk patients with sustained "mild" uncomplicated hypertension (diastolic BP 90-109 mmHg) for 10 years to prevent one stroke, MI or death).

In order to target treatment of high BP appropriately, the BHS has adopted a treatment threshold of absolute level of risk of coronary heart disease of 1.5% per year (i.e. roughly 15% over 10 years), equivalent to a 20% 10 year risk of developing any cardiovascular event. In other words, if 100 people at this level of risk were observed over 10 years, 85 would be free of a CHD event at the end. This number would be increased to approximately 89 if all patients received a treatment reducing relative risk by 25%. Absolute individual CHD risk can be estimated using tables (e.g. the Joint British Tables - see Chapter 4) developed for this purpose. To use these, one needs to know simple data such as age, gender, smoker (yes/ no), diabetes (yes/ no), and total: HDL cholesterol ratio – and of course BP (pre-treatment if possible).

Even when measured properly (which is not always the case), BP varies over time and according to the context in which it is measured. It also responds variably to non-pharmacological interventions. Therefore, when mildly elevated BP (>140/90 mmHg) is detected opportunistically, arrangements should be made to repeat measurements monthly for 4-6 months. This is to avoid making inappropriate decisions on lifelong drug treatment. Non-pharmacological advice (see below) should be given at this stage. Wherever possible, the patient should be prompted to return for further measurements.

- **Assessment - "who to treat?"**

Aims to determine:

1) risk factors for stroke and MI other than hypertension
2) presence of existing target organ damage or cardiovascular complications
3) the likelihood of a secondary cause
4) coexisting conditions which may influence eventual choice of therapy
5) therapy which previously has been ineffective or poorly tolerated
6) exacerbating factors

Thus:

History: smoking status (current or ex-smoker), diet (salt, alcohol), personal history of asthma/gout/MI/stroke, family history of vascular disease

Examination: general appearance, weight (body mass index), bruits, palpable kidneys, peripheral pulses, retinopathy

Investigations: urinalysis, electrolytes and blood glucose, serum lipids (total and HDL cholesterol, and triglycerides), ECG

If BP settles over this period, it should be rechecked annually (Figure 1). If it does not, it is important to determine whether the individual in question has an absolute cardiovascular risk of ≥2%/year. If BP remains at ≥140/90 mmHg (either systolic or diastolic), it should be treated in those who have a high absolute cardiovascular risk for whatever reason. This will include older patients (>60 years) and those with target organ damage/cardiovascular complications, and those identified by the tables. Otherwise, it should be reassessed annually.

In those with a higher BP at detection (≥160/100 mmHg), exactly the same assessments should be performed. BP will settle considerably in some individuals. If there is target organ damage or a history of cardiovascular complications, antihypertensive therapy should be started if BP remains at these levels after one month. Formal evaluation of cardiovascular risk is less critical to antihypertensive decision-making as the benefits of treatment are clear-cut at these BP levels. In those without target organ damage, therapy should begin if the same level of BP is observed over a period of three months. If BP falls to the range 140-160/90-100 mmHg, it should be assessed as above in the context of absolute risk.

In more severe cases, (BP is ≥220/110 mmHg) at detection, treatment should be started immediately. If it is ≥200/100mmHg, the period of assessment should be only two weeks.

Target BP: Aim for a systolic blood pressure < 140 mm Hg and a diastolic blood pressure of <85 mmHg. A lower target (<80 mmHg) should be used in people with diabetes (HOT study).

- **Non-pharmacological therapy**
  This can be tailored according to lifestyle. Family doctors are only too aware that imparting information is often an ineffective way of changing behavior. However, change is dependent on doctor as well as patient factors and is more likely when a

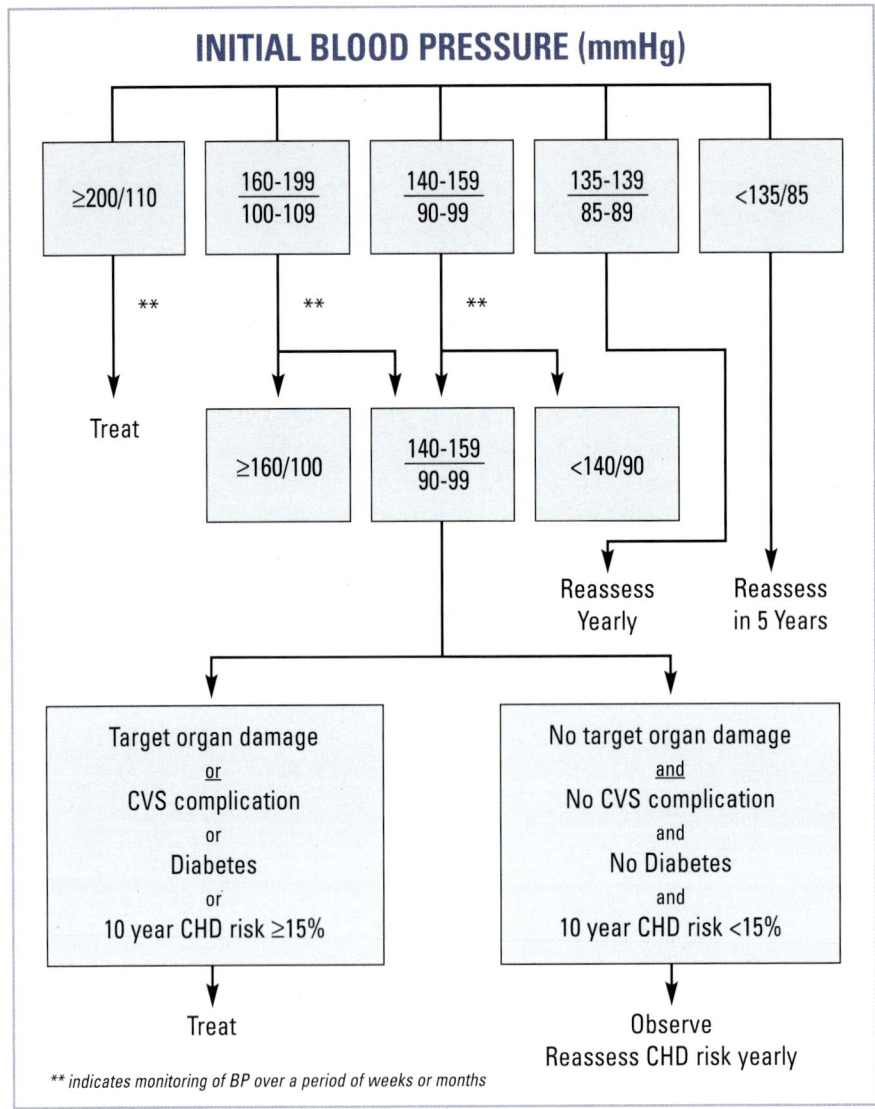

Figure 1. British Hypertension Society guidelines for management of hypertension

relationship has developed and been maintained over a period of time. It may be best to focus on one change at a time (starting with number (1)):

1) Stop smoking: the cardiovascular benefits far outweigh those of treatment of mild hypertension (and the risks associated with any weight gain).

2) Reduce salt intake: half salt intake by not adding salt and avoiding "ready" meals (aim for < 100 mmol sodium per day). This may enhance the response to drug treatment, especially ACE inhibitors.

3) Weight management: diet and exercise lower blood pressure. Supervision by a dietician should aim at modest and sustained weight loss via education and positive changes in lifestyle choices. Every 1 kg reduction in weight causes about a 1 mm Hg reduction in obese hypertensives, as shown in the Nurses' Health Study in the USA.

4) Limit alcohol consumption to 10 units for men and 7 units for women per week.

5) Improve diet: More fruit, less saturated fat and sugar.

In the longer term, changes in lifestyle will be achieved via health promotion at a population level and/or regulatory action.

Pharmacological therapy

Six main classes of drug are currently prescribed (see Introductory Chapter for details); other agents are emerging continually. All are effective in reducing blood pressure (by different mechanisms) and have now been shown either to improve outcome compared with placebo, or to have an equivalent effect on cardiovascular mortality to that of more established classes. There are no robust randomized data to date to implicate definite superiority of one class of drug over another, except angiotensin receptor blockers over beta blockers in patients with LVH. Most doctors have preferred "first-line" agents according to particular patient characteristics, but finding the right agent(s) for an individual is often a process of trial and error. Only half of all patients will be controlled on one drug and many require two or three agents to achieve targets.

Thiazide diuretics: Bendrofluazide is the cheapest agent and is effective in preventing stroke and MI particularly in the elderly (and in black patients). In the lowest available dose (2.5 mg), it causes little disturbance of blood lipids but should be avoided in patients with severe dyslipidemia. Erectile dysfunction is reported by some patients. Some elderly patients develop severe hyponatremia as a rare and unpredictable reaction which responds promptly to withdrawal. In spite of causing slight increases in blood sugar, bendrofluazide is effective in preventing MI in patients with type 2 diabetes and is highly effective in combination with an ACE inhibitor. Loop diuretics (e.g. frusemide) are more effective in terms of BP lowering than thiazides in patients with impaired renal function.

The ALLHAT trial

The importance of thiazide diuretics has recently been underlined by the publication in December 2002 of the American ALLHAT study. ALLHAT studied 33,357 hypertensive patients, randomized to the thiazide chlorthalidone, lisinopril or amlodipine. The mean age was 67 and 47% were women. 35% were black and 19% were Hispanic. After 4.9 years of follow-up it was seen that the three drugs were equally good at preventing fatal or non fatal cardiac death or MI, the primary end point of the trial.

The thiazide lowered systolic blood pressure slightly more than the other two. There were fewer heart failure cases with chlorthalidone than with Amlodipine, and surprisingly, fewer with chlorthalidone than with lisinopril. Overall mortality was not different between the groups. A fourth group on doxazosin was discontinued early because of an excess of heart failure compared to chlorthalidone. Disappointingly there was not a beta blocker group, and beta blockers were available as second line across all the groups.

Nevertheless, ALLHAT shows that for uncomplicated hypertensive patients thiazides have a valuable role. In the light of ALLHAT support for these cheaper agents has been resurgent.

ß-blockers: These agents (e.g. atenolol) are relatively cheap and are proven to prevent stroke and (to a lesser extent) MI. They are particularly useful in younger patients, anxious patients and those with angina or a past history of MI. They cannot be used in patients with asthma (bronchoconstriction), poorly-controlled insulin-treated diabetics (hypoglacemia), heart block (bradycardia), or clinically significant peripheral vascular disease (claudication). In addition, their use is limited by more subtle adverse effects such as fatigue, nightmares and impaired concentration.

Calcium-channel blockers: There are three subclasses of these more expensive agents: one member of the dihydropyridine subclass (nitrendipine) has been shown to reduce stroke and MI in older patients. Most doctors are more familiar with its sister drug nifedipine. Use of short-acting preparations, previously recommended for management of hypertensive emergencies, may be dangerous; long-acting preparations (Amlodipine; nifedipine GITS, Nifedipine, once daily modified release preparation) are now preferred. Mild facial flushing occurs (usually transiently) in some patients; ankle edema occurs in 5-10% and is the most common reason for discontinuing therapy. Cousins from the other subclasses (verapamil and diltiazem) are also effective agents. They are more frequently used in patients with angina and should not be co-prescribed with ß-blockers as they may cause severe bradycardia. Claims that calcium channel blockers cause increased mortality in patients with diabetes have not been substantiated.

ACE inhibitors: There are fewer outcome data with these agents in hypertension (e.g. enalapril, fosinopril, lisinopril, perindopril, ramipril, trandolapril), although there are abundant data for heart failure. At the time of their introduction it was considered unethical to compare them with placebo and, after some delay, three large studies comparing them with traditional agents evolved, ALLHAT (see above), ASCOT and ANBP2 (still in progress).

The HOPE trial, which compared ramipril with placebo showed important gains, likely caused by lowering blood pressure and blockade of the renin-angiotensin system. In a recently-published long-term UK trial in hypertensive patients with diabetes (UKPDS), one of the earliest members of this class (captopril) appeared to have similar efficacy to atenolol in preventing stroke, although the study was underpowered to demonstrate equivalence formally.

ACE inhibitors are well tolerated and effective in patients who have experienced adverse effects on other agents. They should be used with extreme caution in women of reproductive age; treatment should stop in those who develop dry cough (10%) or angio-edema (rare). A further difficulty with their use in a non-specialist setting is that a small proportion of patients who have unsuspected bilateral renal artery stenosis develop acute renal failure requiring hemodialysis (caution: young patients, rapid onset of severe hypertension, refractory disease, abdominal bruits, raised creatinine). This can be prevented by careful monitoring of urea and electrolytes at the start of therapy.

Angiotensin II receptor blockers: Losartan, candesartan, valsartan, irbesartan and others are the newest class of drugs to have persuasive evidence. They block the action of angiotensin II at its receptor, just as ß-blockers block catecholamines at beta adrenoceptors. Proven in patients with LVH, and in people with diabetes with frank nephropathy, they have a very favorable side effect profile. ARBs are being used increasingly as first line therapy. They have no effect on bradykinin and therefore do not cause cough, hence are useful in patients who develop cough on ACE inhibitors. Recently, losartan-based therapy has been shown to have considerable superiority over atenolol-based therapy in patients with hypertension and left ventricular hypertrophy in the LIFE study. Benefits were especially marked in diabetics and in patients with systolic hypertension.

Other drugs:

Aspirin: Although it does not lower blood pressure, aspirin is effective in preventing myocardial infarction in well-controlled hypertensive patients over 50 years old who have target organ damage/cardiovascular complications or an absolute cardiovascular risk of ≥2% per year.

Alpha-blockers: Doxazosin may be added in for patients who are poorly controlled on other agents and is useful in patients with renal failure. It is effective in lowering blood pressure, but is associated with a higher incidence of heart failure than low dose diuretic therapy. It is usually co-prescribed with a diuretic.

Centrally-acting agents: Moxonidine is a recent addition.

Methlydopa: Now mainly used in pregnancy.

Loop diuretics: These are useful in patients with chronic renal failure, when thiazides start to fail as the creatinine rises and tubular function deteriorates.
As a rule of thumb, all patients who are difficult to control on two agents should be assessed at a specialist clinic.

Statins: These drugs have transformed cardiovascular medicine, and are discussed fully in Chapter 4.

Key points
- Absolute cardiovascular risk should be assessed as a basis for treatment decisions

- Systolic blood pressure is a better predictor of risk, except in young or pregnant individuals

- Advantages of treatment are small in low risk people and the decision to start lifelong therapy should not be rushed

- Good management requires excellent local systems of communication amongst patients, family doctors, and hospital specialists.

Further reading:
- **British Hypertension Society Guidelines (third working party).** Journal of Human Hypertension (Nature) 1999; 13: 569-592 (www.hyp.ac.uk/bhsinfo/1000917.pdf)

- **ABC of hypertension.** Gareth Beevers, Gregory Y H Lip, and Eoin O'Brien BMJ 2001; 322: (series).

- **Scottish Intercollegiate Guidelines Network (40).** Lipids and the Primary Prevention of CHD. Edinburgh, Royal College of Physicians, 1999 (http://www.sign.ac.uk/pdf/sign40.pdf)

- **ALLHAT Collaborative Group.** Major outcomes in high-risk hypertensive patients randomized to ACE inhibitor or calcium channel blocker vs diuretic: the Antihypertensive and Lipid Lowering Treatment to prevent Heart Attack Trial (ALLHAT). JAMA 2002;287:2981-2997.

CHAPTER 4

HYPERTENSION, HYPERLIPIDEMIA AND ESTIMATION OF CARDIOVASCULAR RISK
Alison Lee, Mark Davis and Adrian Brady

Key points

● Hyperlipidemia is a major risk factor for cardiovascular disease.

● Combination of risk factors multiply cardiovascular risk.

● Lifestyle changes are the cornerstone of therapy.

● Robust mortality data supports the use of statin therapy in primary and secondary prevention in all groups.

● Guidelines are available for primary prevention; these allow for the calculation of absolute risk of a cardiovascular event for that individual, based on their overall risk profile.

● In primary prevention screening of all patients with hypertension is appropriate, and following calculation of individual risk, lifestyle changes should be advised to reduce risk, in particular cessation of smoking. If the individual has high residual risk, drug treatment for cholesterol should be considered.

Introduction
Hyperlipidemia, hypertension, and smoking are the three most significant remediable risk factors for cardiovascular disease.

Cholesterol And Lipoprotein Metabolism
Cholesterol is essential for cellular membranes, and is largely synthesized by the liver. Dietary fats are formed into chylomicrons in the intestines which circulate to the liver; here the lipids are processed into VLDL (very low density lipoprotein) particles. In the

peripheral tissues triglycerides are cleaved for cellular metabolism. The resultant particles are metabolized by the liver to LDL (low density lipoproteins), which is the major cholesterol carrying moiety. HDL is the other cholesterol rich particle and scavenges free cholesterol released from LDLs. LDL is usually a derived value which is calculated from the following Friedewald equation LDL = Total cholesterol - (HDL+[Triglycerides/2.66]), the results are in mmol/L. The calculation is valid for triglyceride values less than 4.0 mmol/L beyond which the calculation becomes inaccurate. Conversion from mg/dl to mmol/L for cholesterol fractions is achieved by multiplying mg/dl by 0.02586, and for triglycerides by 0.01129.

Cholesterol and Cardiovascular risk
Elevated lipoproteins are commonly due to combination of dietary and genetic factors, however "secondary" causes of hyperlipidemia should be considered, such as diabetes, alcoholism, thyroid disease, liver or renal failure. Initial assessment of lipoproteins should routinely involve checking for secondary causes. Cardiovascular risk correlates directly with total cholesterol, and with LDL cholesterol, but inversely with HDL cholesterol. Alternatively, risk is often assessed using the ratio between total and HDL cholesterol, lower risk being associated with total cholesterol : HDL ratio <5.

Triglycerides are a risk factor for cardiovascular mortality, and can be modified both by diet and medication. However when other epidemiological data are corrected for, e.g. glucose, total cholesterol and HDL, triglycerides become less important. The most recent USA guidelines suggest that with trigycerides below 2.4mmol/L should be treated with diet, and only above this do they become a target for therapy[1].

In determining lipoprotein levels, a fasting sample is not essential for the measurement of total cholesterol, but triglyceride levels can only accurately be assessed after a twelve hour fast. In practice, decisions regarding therapy for both primary and secondary prevention are routinely based on the total cholesterol, or the total cholesterol: HDL ratio which can be assessed on a non fasted sample. Triglycerides in excess of 4.00 mmol/L will interfere with the calculation of LDL hence at least one measurement should be fasted. Provided the triglycerides are low follow-up cholesterol levels can be done unfasted.

The Evidence For Lipid Lowering
There are seven major trials of HMG Co A reductase inhibitors (statins) which show overwhelmingly that lowering cholesterol improves mortality and morbidity from cardiovascular disease. Earlier trials of fibrate drugs did not show overall mortality benefits.

Primary Prevention
The WOSCOPS [2] study looked at 6595 men with moderate cardiovascular risk, but no previous myocardial infarction. They were randomized to pravastatin or placebo, with mean follow-up of 4.9 years. Average baseline total cholesterol was 7 mmol/L, with 20% reduction in the treatment group. Overall risk reduction was 22% for all cause mortality, 33% in death from coronary events, and 31% reduction in non-fatal MI with little effect

on stroke. This was the first primary prevention trial that was adequately powered for mortality end-points.

The American AFCAPS/TEXCAPS study examined a lower risk group that included women[3]. Again, an important 37% reduction in the relative risk of a cardiovascular event was achieved with statin therapy.

However the *absolute* risk of an event in both groups was small, hence the overall benefit of lowering cholesterol in an entire population, most of whom are at a low absolute risk, with statin therapy is not yet economic or necessary. Targeting statin therapy towards those with overall higher absolute risk, is the present strategy in primary prevention.

The Heart Protection Study [4]
This very large study of 20,536 UK adults with existing coronary disease or other atherosclerotic vascular disease, or multiple risk factors deserves special mention. The patients were a mixture of primary and secondary prevention individuals. The results were spectacular. Regardless of patient subtype, presence of DM, age or starting cholesterol level, simvastatin 40 mg treatment for five years substantially reduced total mortality, cardiovascular events and ischemic stroke. This is the strongest argument for lowering cholesterol in everyone at increased risk of CHD.

Secondary Prevention
The 4S trial [5] was the first landmark study to address cholesterol lowering post MI, using Simvastatin against placebo for a follow-up of 5.4 years. The 4S trial studied 4444 Scandinavian men who had had either a myocardial infarction, or unstable angina. There was a mean 25% reduction in total cholesterol, and follow-up demonstrated an overall 30% reduction in mortality in the treatment group, and 37% reduction in non fatal myocardial infarction. Patients with diabetes in particular benefited.

The CARE[6] and the LIPID[7] megatrials also looked at secondary prevention with statin therapy in a lower risk population and confirmed similar reductions in mortality and morbidity.

There is now data on over 40,000 patients prevention studies making an inviolable case for lipid lowering with statin therapy. There is a little data for older drugs, e.g. fibrates which are now used as an adjunct to statin therapy in patients with extreme levels of hyperlipidemia or isolated hypertriglyceridemia.

The recently published PROSPER trial[8] studied an elderly population at high risk of stroke. Disappointingly, over a three year follow-up period stroke and incidence of dementia were not reduced, although cardiac events decreased. A longer period of follow might have been successful, since the HPS study showed the benefit against stroke was principally over long term therapy.

Therapy In Hyperlipidemia

Lifestyle: A reduced saturated fat diet is the basis for treatment of hyperlipidemia, and dietary advice to encourage weight loss and improve the ratio between HDL and total cholesterol is mandatory for treatment of all hyperlipidemic patients especially if hypertensive. Exercise will also improve the ratio between total cholesterol and HDL. With good dietary compliance of a reduced fat diet a mean reduction of between 5 and 9% in total cholesterol can be achieved[7], although there is marked inter-individual variation. Liaison with a dietician for advice and encouragement is helpful, although may not be readily available, and specific diets are in the literature.

Even simple dietary advice such as increased intake of fruit and vegetables, alterations in cooking methods e.g. reduced fried food, alcohol and sugar can help. More recently modified margarine containing either natural or synthetic plant stanols or sterols, have been shown to lower both total and LDL cholesterol by about 10% in a dose dependent manner[9]).

There is now an extensive and growing literature on the effects of dietary intervention with plant sterol enriched margarine. Clinically the basis of all therapy in hyperlipidemia, particularly in those with concomitant hypertension, is diet and lifestyle modification. If the individuals absolute risk is unacceptably high as assessed using the available charts discussed below then drug therapy should be considered. The HPS study is a powerful argument for statin treatment earlier rather than later.

Drug Treatment
Drug treatment is divided into those drugs exerting a primary effect on total and LDL cholesterol, or on triglycerides.

Cholesterol lowering

Statins (HMG CoA Reductase inhibitors): These drugs inhibit the rate limiting step in cholesterol synthesis in the liver. Therapy reduces total cholesterol by 30% at standard dose, with 10% reduction in triglycerides, and improvements in total cholesterol: HDL ratio[2]. In the latest trials high dose statins can be shown to reduce cholesterol by up to 50%, and we routinely use high doses. Therapy is well tolerated, with the incidence of side effects in the major trials being comparable to placebo[2]. The main side effects reported are myositis, asymptomatic elevation of liver and muscle enzymes, and gastrointestinal upset. There is now ten years of safety data on some of the statins, which are effective and remarkably safe drugs, despite powerful actions on liver metabolism.

Anion exchange resins: These act to bind bile acids in the gut, causing reduced re-circulation of bile acids, and increased removal of LDL from the circulation.

Cholestyramine is the only commonly used member, and can reduce LDL by 20% although triglycerides increase[9]. Side effects are common, including bloating, flatulence, and constipation, so few tolerate more than two sachets/day.

Ezetimibe: This new drug specifically inhibits cholesterol absorption in the GI tract. It will probably be used mostly as an adjunct to statin therapy, lowering LDL by a useful additional margin.

Triglyceride Lowering

Fibric acid derivatives: These drugs reduce triglycerides by around 50%, and have varying effects on total and LDL cholesterol depending on the baseline profile, however they tend to increase HDL[10]. They have similar side effect profile to the statins.

Nicotinic acid: This parent compound is now rarely used because of side effects, severe flushing and gastrointestinal upset, but does reduce both triglycerides, and cholesterol. Two derivatives are available, Acipimox, and Nitrofurandole, which have fewer side effects and are slightly less potent.

Other drugs are available, such as Probucol, but its use is rare.
Omega 3 fatty acids are emerging in this area with important anti-arrhythmic properties.

Interaction With Anti Hypertensive Agents

Few of the modern anti hypertensive agents interact with serum cholesterol, and selection of anti-hypertensive should not be affected by lipid level. ACE inhibitors, calcium channel antagonists, and hydralazine are all lipid neutral. Classically, thiazide diuretics can cause minor increases in LDL (mean increase 0.25mmol/L) and triglycerides, with no effect on HDL[10]. Loop diuretics have similar effects but can also reduce HDL. ß-blockers may increase triglycerides, and lower HDL, and α-blockers have a beneficial effect on lipids. However we believe that adequate lowering of blood pressure is crucial in this group and effective anti-hypertensives should not be avoided because of trivial effects on blood lipids. For example, while many lipid neutral drugs are available, principally vasodilators, many of these need a diuretic for maximum effect.

Millions of patients receive concomitant statins and antihypertensive therapy without problem. Cholestyramine can affect absorption of other medicines, in particular ß-blockers and thiazides, and should be taken at a different time. Nicotinic acid can exaggerate the blood pressure lowering effect of vasodilators, and these drugs should be used with caution in combination.

Who to Treat?

Secondary Prevention

Treating cholesterol in those with established ischemic heart disease is now accepted, the questions now being asked are

- do all subgroups benefit equally?

- at what level should treatment be started?

- what is the target level?

All patients with coronary disease should be on statins. The evidence is overwhelming, at least up to age 80. Probably most diabetics should too, although this is less well implemented.

Most of the major post infarct trials have smaller proportions of female, diabetic and hypertensive patients, however they show benefit in all sub-groups, including those over 65 years of age [4]. Diabetics in particular benefit, as coronary disease is often more diffuse in this group, and statin therapy is an important adjunct to medical therapy and post coronary bypass surgery.

In Britain, common practice used to use 5.0 mmol/L as the figure above which therapy should be instigated, with a reduction of 30% in total or LDL cholesterol achieved. Now, we start every patient with atheromatous disease on statin therapy, and aim for a substantial fall in cholesterol. In practice this means that British doctors are encouraged to keep the total cholesterol level of their ischemic heart disease patients below 5.0 mmol/L using drug and dietary intervention, the American guidelines however suggest an LDL of 2.5mmol/L, which equates to a total cholesterol around 4.0mmol/L [1]. It is likely that the UK guidelines will become more stringent soon.

Primary Prevention

There are now multiple guidelines published to help identify patients with a high risk profile. Most guidelines accept that hypertension is an indication for lipid screening in an individual. We describe two different guidelines. Clinicians should familiarize themselves with their national or chosen international guideline and use it regularly in primary prevention.

Probably the most commonly used risk evaluation tables in the UK are derived from the Joint British recommendations on prevention of coronary heart disease in clinical practice [11]. These tables are widely available and in addition are published as appendices in the British National Formulary (See Figures 1 and 2 below). To use these, the correct chart is identified for the individual as they are subdivided into males and females, diabetics and non diabetics, smokers and non-smokers.

The subjects' total cholesterol to HDL cholesterol ratio is calculated using the nomogram on the top right corner. The cholesterol ratio and systolic blood pressure are then used to plot the individual on the chart and the 10 year risk can be derived. These charts are easy to use, although they underestimate risk in British Asians and in those with very high triglycerides. In general, drug treatment is recommended for those with a 30% or greater risk over 10 years, a level set for financial rather than medical reasons. This 30% figure may soon change.

The most recent guidelines to be published are the American guidelines, which are reported by the National Cholesterol Education Program (NCEP) in their third report[1]. The American guidelines suggest that all subjects over the age of twenty should be tested five yearly with a full fasted lipoprotein screen. The individuals are then subdivided into degree of risk, with highest risk category being those with known coronary heart disease, secondly those with multiple risk factors, and thirdly those with less than two risk major risk factors.

In their assessment, the presence of diabetes confers a similar risk to the presence of known coronary heart disease therefore the five identified risk factors are smoking, hypertension, low HDL cholesterol, age (>45yrs in men >55yrs in women), and premature coronary heart disease in a first degree relative. If the subject is in the highest risk category, i.e. with known CHD or diabetes, then lifestyle and drug therapy should achieve a LDL cholesterol of 2.5mmol/L (100mg/dL).

If the individual is in the multiple risk factor group, the Framingham data is used to assess the risk on a points scoring basis (Appendix 3). Points are given for the individual's level of each risk factor, then summed, and the bottom table establishes 10 year risk. Where risk using this data is 10-20% in ten years, the guidelines state that LDL should be below 3.4mmol/L, using diet and drugs. If however the calculated risk is <10% in ten years, then a higher LDL of 4.1 mmol/L is accepted before drugs are introduced. If the individual has less than two risks, then the LDL goal is 4.1mmol/L, above which diet is considered, and drug therapy should be used if the LDL despite diet remains above 4.9mmol/L.

Conclusion

Data are now available that risk factors multiply in individuals. The hypertensive patient with high blood lipids is at higher risk of cardiovascular events, and all hypertensive patients should have lipid screening done and lifestyle advice given. In primary prevention there are several useful tables that can be used to assess individual risk over the next years, and it is recommended that physicians become familiar with one table for risk stratification and introduction of therapy. All patients with established coronary heart disease, either angina or myocardial infarction, should have cholesterol below 5.0 mmol/L. If statin therapy is required to achieve this then it should be used. Statin therapy may soon be standard therapy for most diabetics.

Priority for treatment therefore is post MI patients, followed by those with overt atherosclerosis, and diabetics and thirdly those with an adverse risk profile in primary prevention.

References

1. Executive summary of the Third Report of the National Cholesterol Education Programe (NCEP) Expert panel on detection, evaluation, and treatment of high blood cholesterol in adults (Adult Treatment Panel III). *JAMA* 2001; 19: 2486-2497.

2. Shepherd J, Cobbe SM, Ford I, et al for the West of Scotland Coronary Prevention Study group. Prevention of coronary heart disease with Pravastatin in men with hypercholesterolemia. *N Engl J Med* 1995; 333: 1301-1307.

3. Downs JR, Clearfield M, Weis S, et al, for the AFCAPS/TEXCAPS Research Group. Primary prevention of acute coronary events with lovastatin in men and women with average cholesterol levels. *JAMA* 1998; 279: 1615-1622.

4. Heart Protection Study Collaborative Group. MRC/BHF Heart Protection Study of antioxidant vitamin supplementation in 20,536 high risk individuals: results of a randomised placebo controlled trial. *Lancet* 2002; 360: 23-33.

5. Scandinavian Simvastatin Survival Group. Randomised trial of cholesterol lowering in 4444 patients with coronary heart disease: the Scandinavian Simvastatin Survival Study (4S). *Lancet* 1994; 344: 1383-1389.

6. Sacks FM, Pfeffer MA, Moye LA, et al for the Cholesterol And Recurrent Events trial investigators. The effect of Pravastatin on Coronary Events after myocardial infarction in patients with average cholesterol levels. *N Engl J Med* 1996; 335: 1001-1009.

7. The Long term Intervention with Pravastatin in Ischemic Disease (LIPID) Study Group: Prevention of cardiovascular events and death with Pravastatin in patients with coronary heart disease and a broad range of cholesterol levels. *N Engl J Med* 1998; 339: 1349-1357.

8. Shepherd J, et al. Pravastatin in elderly individuals at risk of vascular disease (PROSPER). *Lancet* 2002;360:1623-1630.

9. Howell WH, McNamara DJ, Tosca MA, Smith BT, Gaines JA. Plasma lipid and lipoprotein responses to dietary fat and cholesterol: a meta analysis. *Am J Clin Nutr* 1997; 65: 1747-1764.

10. Hallikainen MA, Sarkkinen ES, Uusitupa MI. Plant stanol esters affect serum cholesterol concentration of hypercholesterolaemic men and women in a dose dependent manner. *J Nutr* 2000; 130: 767-776.

11. Betteridge DJ, Dodson PM, Durrington PN, Hughes EA, et al. Management of Ilyperlipidaemia: guidelines of the British Hyperlipidaemia Association. *Postgrad Med J* 1993; 69: 359-369.

12. National Cholesterol Education Programme. Second report of the expert panel on detection, evaluation, and treatment of high blood cholesterol in adults. *Circulation* 1994; 89: 1333-1345.

13. Wood D, Durrington P, Poulter N, et al. Joint British recommendations on prevention of coronary heart disease in clinical practice. *Heart* 1998; 80: Supp 2.

14. Haq IU, Jackson PR, Yeo WW, Ramsey LE. Sheffield risk and treatment table for cholesterol lowering for primary prevention of coronary heart disease. *Lancet* 1995; 346: 1467-1471.

Appendix 1a
Estimate of 10-year risk for **Men** (Framingham Point scores).
Reproduced with kind permission from the NHLBI, Bethesda, Maryland, USA.

Age,years	Points
20-34	-9
35-39	-4
40-44	0
45-49	3
50-54	6
55-59	8
60-64	10
65-69	11
70-74	12
75-79	13

Total Cholesterol mg/dL(mmol/L)	Points				
	Age 20-39y	Age 40-49y	Age 50-59y	Age 60-69y	Age 70-79y
<160 (<4.1)	0	0	0	0	0
160-199 (4.1-5.1)	4	3	2	1	0
200-239 (5.1-6.2)	7	5	3	1	0
240-279 (6.2-7.2)	9	6	4	2	1
>280 (>7.2)	11	8	5	3	1

	Points				
	Age 20-39y	Age 40-49y	Age 50-59y	Age 60-69y	Age 70-79y
Nonsmoker	0	0	0	0	0
Smoker	8	5	3	1	1

HDL mg/dl (mmo/L)	Points
>60 (1.5)	-1
50-59 (1.3-1.5)	0
40-49 (1.0-1.3)	1
<40 (<1.0)	2

Systolic BP mmHg	If Untreated	If Treated
<120	0	0
120-129	0	1
130-139	1	2
140-159	1	2
>160	2	3

Points total	10-year risk %
<0	<1
0	1
1	1
2	1
3	1
4	1
5	2
6	2
7	3
8	4
9	5
10	6
11	8
12	10
13	12
14	16
15	20
16	25
> 17	>30

To use the tables identify the appropriate points value for the subject in each risk category, then sum these and use the bottom table to find the calculated ten year risk of a cardiovascular event. Converting mg/dl to mmol/L multiply by 0.02586
Tables modified from the US guidelines published in JAMA 2001; 19: 2486-2497.

Appendix 1b
Estimate of 10-year risk for **Women** (Framingham Point scores).

Age,years	Points
20-34	-7
35-39	-3
40-44	0
45-49	3
50-54	6
55-59	8
60-64	10
65-69	12
70-74	14
75-79	16

Total Cholesterol mg/dL(mmol/L)	Points				
	Age 20-39y	Age 40-49y	Age 50-59y	Age 60-69y	Age 70-79y
<160 (<4.1)	0	0	0	0	0
160-199 (4.1-5.1)	4	3	2	1	1
200-239 (5.1-6.2)	8	6	4	2	1
240-279 (6.2-7.2)	11	8	5	3	2
>280 (>7.2)	13	10	7	4	2

	Points				
	Age 20-39y	Age 40-49y	Age 50-59y	Age 60-69y	Age 70-79y
Nonsmoker	0	0	0	0	0
Smoker	9	7	4	2	1

HDL mg/dl (mmo/L)	Points
>60 (1.5)	-1
50-59 (1.3-1.5)	0
40-49 (1.0-1.3)	1
<40 (<1.0)	2

Systolic BP mmHg	If Untreated	If Treated
<120	0	0
120-129	1	3
130-139	2	4
140-159	3	5
>160	4	6

Points total	10-year risk %
<9	<1
9	1
10	1
11	1
12	1
13	2
14	2
15	3
16	4
17	5
18	6
19	8
20	11
21	14
22	17
23	22
24	27
>25	>30

To use the tables identify the appropriate points value for the subject in each risk category, then sum these and use the bottom table to find the calculated ten year risk of a cardiovascular event. Converting mg/dl to mmol/L multiply by 0.02586 Tables modified from the US guidelines published in JAMA 2001; 19: 2486-2497.

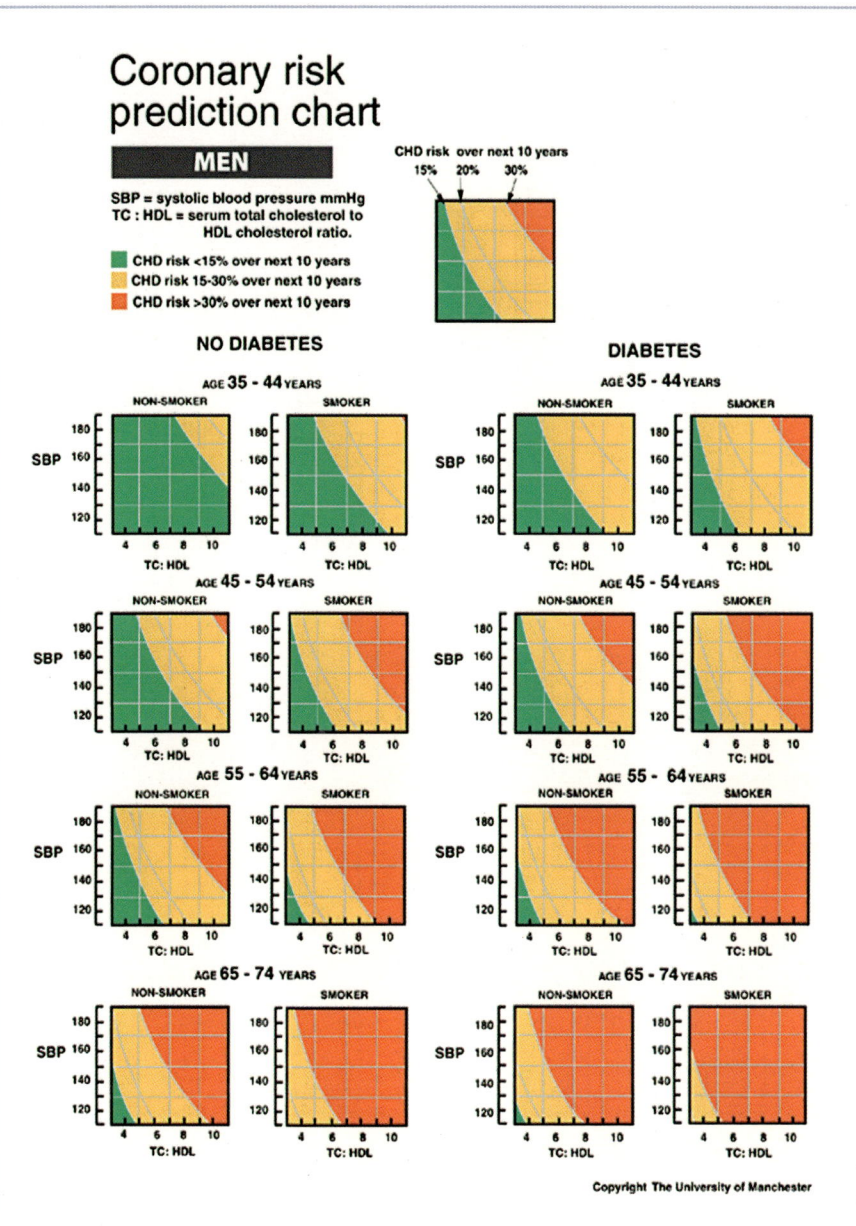

Figure 1. *Joint British Guidelines for the Primary Prevention of Coronary Heart Disease (men).*

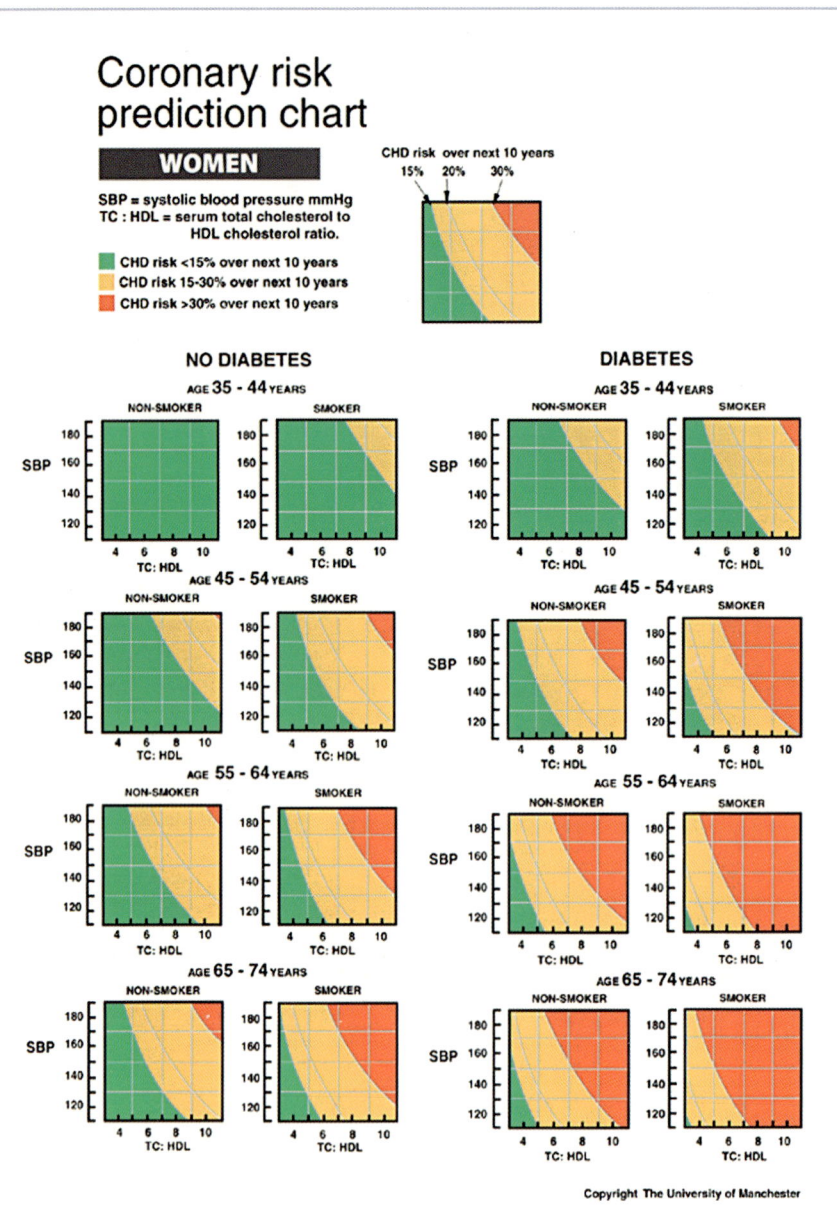

*Figure 2. Joint British Guidelines for the Primary Prevention of Coronary Heart Disease (women)
Reproduced with kind permission of the authors and the University of Manchester.*

Table 1: Priorities for Coronary Heart Disease Prevention. (European Guidelines)[9]

1. Patients with established CHD or atherosclerotic vascular disease.
2. Asymptomatic subjects with particularly high risk
3. Close relatives of :
    patients with early onset CHD or other atherosclerotic vascular disease;
    asymptomatic subjects with particularly high risk
4. Other individuals met in connection with ordinary clinical practice.

Table 2: Risk factors for cholesterol lowering. (American Guidelines)[4]

Age->55years for women, >45years for men
Family history of premature vascular disease.
Cigarette smoking
Hypertension
Diabetes mellitus
HDL cholesterol<0.9mmol/L, note that HDL>1.55mmol/L negates one of the other risk factors.

Table 3: Treatment decisions based on LDL cholesterol USA guidelines [4]

	Initiation level mmol/L	Target LDL mmol/L
Dietary therapy		
LOW RISK: without CHD and < 2 risk factors	≥4.1	<4.1
MODERATE RISK: Without CHD and >2 risk factors	≥3.4	<3.4
HIGH RISK: Previous CHD	>2.6	≤ 2.6
Drug treatment		
LOW RISK: without CHD and < 2 risk factors	≥4.9	<4.1
MODERATE RISK: Without CHD and >2 risk factors	≥4.1	<3.4
HIGH RISK: Previous CHD	>3.4	≤ 2.6

CHAPTER 5

LEFT VENTRICULAR HYPERTROPHY IN HYPERTENSION

Neeraj Prasad, Peter Clarkson and Adrian Brady

Introduction

Sir Richard Bright reported in 1836 that the majority who died of glomerulonephritis had large hearts proposing that cardiac enlargement was secondary to increased vascular resistance produced by the distorted blood vessel. In 1914 Lewis reported that raised blood pressure was the most potent factor to produce left ventricular hypertrophy (LVH) compared to valvular disease and renal disease. Left ventricular hypertrophy is a now recognized as a common feature of cardiovascular disease. It is often thought to be a major mechanism of the cardiac adaptation to hemodynamic overload on the heart or contractile failure of the myocardium. LVH is not just an incidental compensatory feature in the evolution of cardiovascular disease but is in fact an ominous predictor of future serious cardiovascular events. It is difficult, however, to define a value of left ventricular mass that separates normal values from pathological hypertrophy. Physiological hypertrophy also occurs, in response to aerobic conditioning exercise. This form of LVH does not demonstrate the same pathophysiological abnormalities as pathological LVH. In pathological LVH there is a disproportionate increase in the mass and volume of the interstitium consisting of fibroblasts and collagen which is not present in physiological LVH and it is this fibroblast growth and deposition of collagen which is thought to be responsible for many of the clinical problems associated with pathological LVH.

Etiology

The chief determinants of LVH in the general population are hypertension, increasing age and obesity although glucose intolerance, alcohol intake, valvular disease and coronary artery disease have a smaller role [1,2]. Unlike the infant heart where hyperplasia of myocytes (increase cell numbers) accounts for cardiac enlargement, in the adult heart hypertrophy of myocytes (an increase in cell size rather than numbers) and increased interstium accounts for ventricular hypertrophy. The basic signals that initiate and maintain myocyte growth include a number of trophic factors. Hypertrophy occurs due to a number of trophic factors (a) hemodynamic factors which cause stretch and deformation either physiological or pathological (eg hypertension, aortic stenosis, coarctation of the aorta),

(b) neurohumerol stimuli (possible roles for the sympathetic system and the renin-angiotensin system), and (c) other stimuli (eg growth hormone, thyroxin, parathyroid hormone, anabolic steroids), including a genetic predisposition. It is not yet completely clear how these trophic factors induce myocyte protein synthesis nor is it completely clear with respect to their relative importance in vivo.

In hypertension, LVH is related to both systolic and diastolic blood pressure but systolic pressure is a better predictor of LV mass. Single resting blood pressure correlates to LV mass however 24-hour blood pressure readings correlate more closely than clinic readings. Twenty four hour blood pressure is not the sole factor for the development of LVH.

Angiotensin II and aldosterone are likely to be trophic factor as much has been reported about their property to stimulate DNA, RNA and protein synthesis with myocardial cell growth as well as increases in the interstitium (via fibroblast growth and collagen deposition)[3]. Additionally, angiotensin II acts as a positive inotrope directly and indirectly by the release of catecholamines from nerve endings which is a further stimuli to hypertrophy.

Prevalence of left ventricular hypertrophy
Population studies performed in Framingham have estimated the prevalence in the general population of echocardiographically determined LVH (Echo-LVH) to be 16% in males and 19% in females[1], and the prevalence of electrocardiographically determined LVH (ECG-LVH) to be about 2-3%[2] ECG-LVH is less sensitive and specific than Echo-LVH, because it represents electromotive vectors generated by the heart rather than directly measuring the bulk of the heart. The prevalence of LVH increases progressively with age.

In those over 70 years of age, Echo-LVH is present in 48% of women and 30% of men. Obesity is strongly associated with LVH with a 9 and 10 fold increase in women and men respectively in those with the highest body mass index versus those with the lowest body

---

Box 1- Prevalence of LVH

- ECG-LVH is present in 2-3% of the population
- Echo-LVH is present in 16% of males and 19% of females
- Prevalence of LVH increases with age (in over 70 yr olds Echo-LVH is present in 30% of men and 48% of women)
- Obesity is strongly associated with LVH
- Recent reduction in the prevalence of LVH is due to better risk factor control

mass index. A downward secular trend in the prevalence of LVH in the Framingham study has been observed for the past four decades, which is thought to be secondary to better control of the risk factors for the genesis of LVH[4].

Diagnosis of left ventricular hypertrophy

ECG-LVH has been recognized since the demonstration in 1912 by Einthoven that LVH was associated with marked increases in QRS voltages and in 1929 by Barnes that T wave changes occurred in severe hypertension (indicating strain). The current criteria for the diagnosis of ECG-LVH are shown in the table (and in chapter 1). Strain may also be present, which is represented by ST segment depression and T wave flattening or inversion. Standard echocardiographic assessment of left ventricular mass consists of an M-mode echocardiograph being taken from the parasternal view at the level of the mitral valve tips, with measurements of left ventricular internal diameter, ventricular septal thickness and posterior wall thickness taken at end diastole, as defined by the onset of the QRS complex on a simultaneous electrocardiograph.

Box 2- Electrocardiographic criteria for left ventricular hypertrophy

- S wave in V1 plus R wave in V5 or 6 (whichever is greater) > 35mm
- Deepest S wave plus tallest R wave in chest leads > 40mm
- R wave in V4, V5, V6 > 27mm
- S wave in V1, V2, V3, > 30mm
- Net positivity lead I plus net negativity lead 3 > 17mm
- R in aVL lead > 13mm
- R in aVF lead > 20mm

There is no universally accepted upper limit for LV mass, although 134 g/m^2 (indexed to body surface area) in males and 110 g/m^2 in females with measurements made in accordance with the Penn convention are the most commonly used.

Echocardiography has also demonstrated three separate subtypes of LVH:

(a) *concentric hypertrophy* - with increased left ventricular mass, increased wall thickness but unchanged cavity size. This subtype tends to be found in pressure overload and is the predominant form in elderly and middle aged hypertensives.

(b) *eccentric hypertrophy* - with increased left ventricular mass, normal wall thickness but increased cavity size. This subtype is predominantly found in volume overload states but is also found in a minority of elderly hypertensives.

(c) ***ventricular remodeling*** - with normal left ventricular mass, thickened walls and decreased cavity size. The significance of this subtype remains unclear.

LVH as a risk factor

The Framingham heart studies have conclusively demonstrated that ECG-LVH is a powerful independent predictor of future mortality and morbidity from cardiovascular disease and sudden death[4]. An age adjusted excess risk for cardiovascular events of 129 per 1000 was observed in males aged 35-64 years, with ECG-LVH compared with the general population whereas in females, aged 35-64 years, an excess risk of 117 per 1000 was observed. These risks appear even greater in subjects over 65 years of age[5].

Box 3- Risks of LVH

Excess risk associated with ECG-LVH

- congestive cardiac failure 50 per 1000

- stroke 20 per 1000

- sudden death 15 per 1000

- coronary heart disease 50 per 1000

Echo-LVH

- Every 50g/m of LV mass (indexed to height) above normal increases cardiovascular disease risk by a factor of 1.49 in males and 1.57 in females

- Concentric LVH confers a worse prognosis than other forms

When subdivided into separate cardiovascular diseases it was demonstrated that the excess risk of clinical congestive cardiac failure was 50 per 1000, stroke 20 per 1000, sudden death 15 per 1000 and coronary heart disease 50 per 1000 [4].

ECG-LVH is a more potent predictor of future cardiovascular events than blood pressure (from which it is an independent risk factor), smoking habita, impaired glucose tolerance or abnormal lipid profile, although it acts synergistically with all of these risk factors to determine the overall level of cardiovascular risk. ECG-LVH is an even more powerful risk factor for future cardiovascular events than the number of stenosed coronary arteries or ejection fraction[6].

Data for Echo-LVH as a risk factor is less extensive than that for ECG-LVH because echocardiography is a relatively newer technique for the investigation of hypertensive heart disease and thus follow up for clinical outcomes is relatively short. However, Echo-LVH has also been demonstrated to be an independent risk factor for cardiovascular events and sudden death. Framingham statistics have demonstrated that, with every 50g/m of left ventricular mass (indexed to height) above the normal range, the risk of cardiovascular disease increased by a factor of 1.49 in males and 1.57 in females[7]. Concentric LVH appears to carry a worse prognosis than other forms. The risk in patients with both ECG-LVH and anatomical LVH is substantially greater than either alone[4].

The main pathological mechanism that relate LVH with cardiovascular morbidity and mortality are postulated to be:

(a) *Ischemic changes;* Myocardial ischemia can result either from perfusion abnormalities in the hypertrophied ventricle (since LVH decreases coronary reserve and impedes myocardial oxygenation) or from associated coronary artery disease.

(b) *Arrhythmias;* ventricular ectopy is increased 40-50 times in patients with LVH than those without[8]. There is also an increase of 10 to 28% of non sustained ventricular tachycardia. The possible mechanism for the arrhythmia altered electrophysiological properties of the hypertrophied myocyte, re-entrant mechanism caused by myocardial fibrosis, myocardial ischemia, LV dysfunction and electrolyte imbalance caused by anti-hypertensive therapy. However, despite the increase of ventricular arrhythmias in LVH, there is no evidence at the moment of sustained ventricular tachycardia and the this increase in ventricular ectopy or non sustained tachycardia is not necessarily a marker for sudden death.

(c) *Impaired diastolic filling;* this is secondary not only to fibrosis which impairs left ventricular compliance, but also impaired myocyte relaxation. The latter may explain the high risk of future development of clinical cardiac failure in those with LVH.

(d) *Impaired myocardial contractility.* In early disease the ventricular systolic function is normal at rest although an abnormal response to exercise has been demonstrated. With long-standing disease dilatation of the left ventricular cavity may occur with reduced resting systolic function.

Regression of LVH
In view of the poor prognosis associated with LVH the efficacy of correcting LVH has recently been subject to intensive investigation. Regression of LVH has been demonstrated following weight reduction in the obese subjects and following salt restriction in hypertensives.

Three large meta-analyses of regression of LVH by anti-hypertensive drug therapy (reviewing 104, 109 and 39 studies respectively) have demonstrated that most forms of antihypertensive therapy are capable of regressing LVH. After correction for the degree of blood pressure lowering angiotensin converting enzyme inhibitors and combination anti-hypertensive therapy probably regress LVH more quickly and more completely than other or single agents. Vasodilator drugs such as hydralazine and minoxidil appear relatively ineffective at reducing LVH, whereas most other agents, fall between these two categories [9,10,11]. In most studies, a significant decrease in LV mass is evident after treatment duration's of three to six months.

These studies have concentrated principally on the regression of left ventricular mass. This tends to imply regression of hypertrophied myocytes since the majority of left ventricular mass is cardiac myocytes. Non-myocyte regression has been less well studied although there is a growing body of evidence that rennin-angiotensin-aldosterone blockade may regress non-myocytes [12].

Some theoretical concern has been voiced about the regression of LVH- with the regression of LVH being primarily due to reduced myocyte volume leaving fibrotic and other supporting tissues unaffected, thus diminished contractile reserve in the presence of a haemodynamic load. If this does occur, then it does not appear to be of clinical importance, with numerous studies demonstrating improvement in a variety of cardiovascular indices following LVH regression, for example:

(a) A reduction in LVH associated arrhythmias has been observed following regression of LVH.

(b) An improvement in left ventricular diastolic filling occurs with LVH regression.

(c) An improvement in cardiac contractility occurs with LVH regression.

The main issue, however, is whether LVH regression improves mortality and morbidity. This has now been addressed in the landmark LIFE trial, presented March 2002 [13]. 9193 patients with hypertension and LVH were randomized to therapy based on the angiotensin receptor blocker (ARB) losartan, or atenolol. Achieved blood pressures were comparable, 144/81 mm Hg in the losartan group and 145/81 in the atenolol group; high doses and combination with diuretics were used. The losartan group did much better over five years of follow up, particularly diabetics and older patients (see Figure 1). There was greater regression of LVH in the ARB group and a large reduction in death and in stroke. This very large reduction in sudden cardiac death over beta blockers is all the more surprising since we have always believed beta blockers to be valuable in preventing sudden cardiac death.

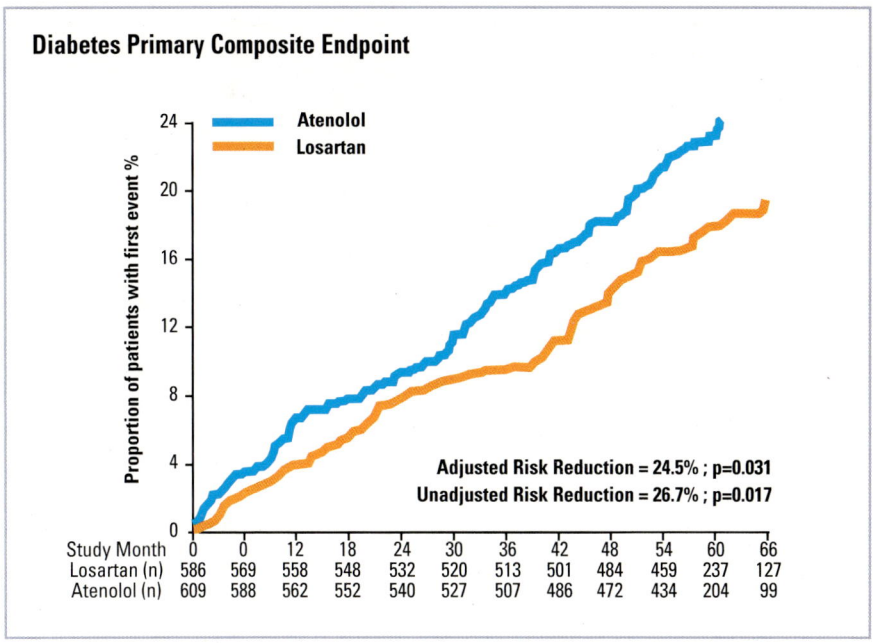

Diabetes Primary Composite Endpoint

Adjusted Risk Reduction = 24.5% ; p=0.031
Unadjusted Risk Reduction = 26.7% ; p=0.017

Study Month	0	0	12	18	24	30	36	42	48	54	60	66
Losartan (n)	586	569	558	548	532	520	513	501	484	459	237	127
Atenolol (n)	609	588	562	552	540	527	507	486	472	434	204	99

Figure 1. LIFE trial: Outcome in patients with hypertension, diabetes and LVH tandomised to atenolol or losartan [13].

Summary

LVH secondary to hypertension is an ominous predictor of future cardiovascular morbidity. Once identified great attention should be taken to normalize the blood pressure. Losartan, (probably other angiotensin receptor blockers) and ACE inhibitors are superior to other classes of drugs and the presence of LVH is an indication for first line therapy with these drugs.

References

1. Levy D, Anderson KM, Savage DD, Kannel WB, Christiansen JC, Castelli WP. Echocardiographically detected left ventricular hypertrophy, prevalence and risk factors. The Framingham Heart Study. *Ann Intern Med* 1988: 108: 2-13.

2. Kannel WB, Dannenberg AL, Levy D. Population implications of ECG left ventricular hypertrophy. *Am J Cardiol* 1987; 60: 851-931.

3. Dzau VJ, Implications of local angiotensin production in cardiovascular physiology and pharmacology. *AM J Cardiol* 1987; 59: 59A-65A.

4. Kannel WB, Cobb J. Left ventricular hypertrophy and mortality - results from the Framingham study. *Cardiology* 1992; 81: 291 -298.

5. Kannel WB. Office assessments of coronary candidates and risk factor insights from the Framingham Study. *J Hypertens* 1991; 9(Suppl &):S13-19.

6. Cooper R, Simmons BE, Castanar A, Santhanam V, Mar M. Left ventricular hypertrophy is associated with increased mortality independent of ventricular function and number of coronary arteries severely narrowed. Am J cardiol 1990; 65: 441-445.

7. Levy D, Garrison RJ, Savage DD, Kannel WB, Castelli WP. Prognostic implications of echocardiographically determined left ventricular mass in the Framingham heart study. *N Engl J med* 1990; 322:1561-6.

8. McLenachan JM, Henderson E, Morris KI, Dargie HJ. Ventricular arrhythmias in patients with hypertensive left ventricular hypertrophy. *N Engl J Med* 1987;317: 787792.

9. Cruickshank JM, Lewis J, Moore V, Dodd C. Reversibility of left ventricular hypertrophy by differing types of antihypertensive therapy. *J Human Hypertens* 1992; 6: 85-90.

10. Dahlof B, Pennert K, Hansson L. Reversal of left ventricular hypertrophy in hypertensive patients. A meta-analysis of 109 treatment studies. *Am J Hypertens* 1992;5 :95-110.

11. Schmieder RE, Martus P, Klingbell A. Reversal of left ventricular hypertrophy in essential hypertention: a metanalysis of randomized double-blind trials. *JAMA* 1996; 275: 1507-1513.

12. Weber KT Brilla CG, Campbell SE, Zhou G, Matsubra L, Guarda E. Pathological hypertrophy with fibrosis: the structural basis for myocardial failure. *Blood pressure* 1992; 1: 75-85.

13. Dahlof B, Devereux RB, et al. Cardiovascular morbidity and mortality in the Losartan for Endpoint reduction in hypertension study. *Lancet* 2002;359:995-1003.

CHAPTER 6

HYPERTENSION IN PATIENTS WITH CONGESTIVE HEART FAILURE *Stuart Hood and Adrian Brady*

The link between heart failure and hypertension

Epidemiological studies have confirmed hypertension as a major risk factor for the development of heart failure. The Framingham study showed that hypertensive individuals had a six-fold-increased risk of developing heart failure compared to normotensives.[1] This relationship holds regardless of age or sex. In addition, the more severe the hypertension, the greater the risk of heart failure. The risk of developing heart failure is more strongly related to the systolic rather than the diastolic blood pressure. It has been estimated that a 10mmHg increase in systolic blood pressure increases the risk of heart failure by 25%.

From hypertension to heart failure

Hypertension is associated with increased peripheral resistance. In turn this causes hypertrophy of the left ventricle (LVH). LVH is accompanied by fibrosis and ultimately reduced contractility of the left ventricle. As heart failure ensues, neurohormonal activation occurs. The sympathetic system is activated early in this disease process and later, activation of the renin-angiotensin system occurs. These neurohormonal abnormalities play a role in the progression of heart failure. Anti-hypertensive drugs, which can alter these neurohormonal changes are therefore a logical choice for the treatment of hypertension in patients with congestive heart failure.

Treatment of hypertension in congestive heart failure patients

Angiotensin converting enzyme (ACE) inhibitors

ACE inhibitors have proven mortality and morbidity benefit in patients with symptomatic or asymptomatic left ventricular (LV) dysfunction.[2] These agents should therefore be prescribed for all hypertensive patients with evidence of LV dysfunction unless there are contraindications. ACE inhibitors will typically reduce mortality by

20-30% and will also reduce the number of hospitalizations for worsening heart failure, myocardial infarction and angina[3]. ACE inhibitors are therefore very cost effective.

Which ACE inhibitor and what dose?

In the treatment of hypertension there are few clinically relevant differences between the ACE inhibitors. All ACE inhibitors are considered equally effective in lowering blood pressure. The recommended doses of ACE inhibitors are the larger doses with proven mortality benefit in clinical trials (e.g. enalapril 10mg bd or captopril 50mg tds).

The ATLAS study compared low dose (2.5-5mg) versus high dose (32.5-35mg) lisinopril. Those taking the higher dose were 12% less likely to die or be hospitalized and 24% less likely to be admitted for heart failure[4]. However, unpublished data from the ATLAS trial suggested that the elderly performed less well with high dose lisinopril. First dose hypotension is unlikely in a hypertensive population. If concerns exist, the first dose can be administered on retiring to bed, or after omitting the morning diuretic dose.

Asymptomatic hypotension occurring after dose escalation does not require withdrawal or dose reduction. Renal function should be monitored after commencing an ACE inhibitor. In practical terms, it is safe to continue ACE inhibitors if creatinine remains <220 µmol/L. Patients should be advised to discontinue ACE-inhibitors in the event of a dehydrating illness as this is a common cause of acute renal failure.

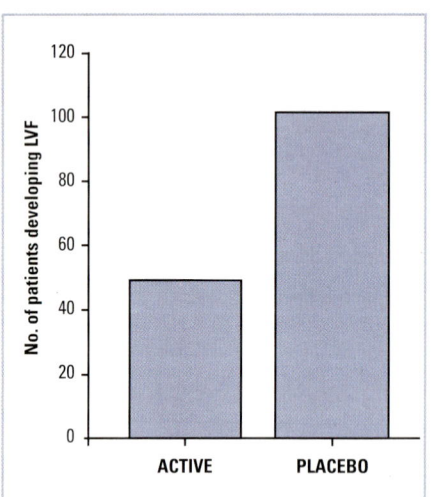

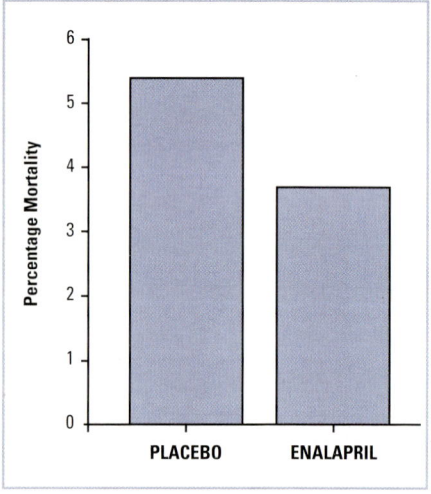

Figure 2. Effects of antihypertensive therapy on the incidence of left ventricular failure (SHEP study [11]).

Figure 3. Three month mortality in the SOLVD study [2].

Diuretics

Thiazide diuretics are a logical choice for the treatment of hypertension in patients with heart failure. Diuretics are very successful in improving heart failure symptoms but no survival data exist. Broadly speaking, diuretics have antihypertensive efficacy similar to other antihypertensives. In practice, however, loop diuretics are often needed for their greater natriuretic effect. Loop diuretics are weaker antihypertensives but are much better for edema. Patients with chronic refigure do not respond to thiazides and loop diuretics in high dose are required.

Recently, the aldosterone antagonist spironolactone has been shown in the RALES trial to confer additional benefit when added to ACE/diuretic combinations. Low doses must be used, and great care must be taken to avoid hyperkalemia when used with ACE inhibitors or ARBs. Our own experience in Glasgow has shown hyperkalemia with these combinations to be commoner than was reported in the RALES trial. Gynecomastia as a side effect is common in men and can limit its use.

Which diuretic and what dose?

The choice of diuretic can be individualized. Thiazide diuretics (e.g. bendrofluazide) generally have a greater antihypertensive effect than loop diuretics (e.g. frusemide). Bendrofluazide, the most commonly used thiazide, has a modest dose response curve over the dose range 1.25-5mg daily. Thiazides tend to be less effective in the presence of renal impairment (GFR< 30-40ml/min) and in this case frusemide may be more suitable. Sometimes a combination of thiazide and loop diuretic may be required for short spells. Patients should weigh themselves 2-3 times weekly as weight gain of 2-3kg might indicate the need to increase diuretic dose. Diuretics usually need to be continued even after edema has resolved, but the dose can be reduced in many cases.

ß-Blockers

ß-blockers are highly effective antihypertensive agents. More recently, the prognostic benefits of ß-blockers in chronic heart failure have been unequivocally proven. Metoprolol, bisoprolol and carvedilol have been shown to improve survival, reduce hospitaliation and improve long-term symptoms of heart failure when given in conjunction with standard anti-failure therapy[5-7]. There is a danger of early symptomatic deterioration however and for this reason, introduction of beta blockade should be undertaken with caution, particularly in patients with severe CHF. General advice is to start at low doses, increasing the dose at 2 weekly intervals ("start low and go slow").

Initial studies of ß-blockers in CHF were confined to patients with mild-moderate heart failure. The more recent COPERNICUS Trial evaluated the effect of carvedilol in patients with severe heart failure (symptoms at rest or minimal exertion).[8]

Carvedilol reduced the risk of death by 35% and the combined endpoint of death or hospitalisation by 24%.

Furthermore, after an acute myocardial infarction complicated by left-ventricular systolic dysfunction, carvedilol reduced the frequency of all-cause and cardiovascular mortality, and recurrent, non-fatal myocardial infarction Capricorn Study)[9]. These beneficial effects were additional to other evidence-based treatments for acute myocardial infarction including ACE inhibitors.

Which ß-blocker and what dose?

Metoprolol, carvedilol and bisoprolol are the evidence-based drugs of choice. Target doses are metoprolol 200mg daily, carvedilol 25-50mg bd and bisoprolol 10 mg daily. In the major heart failure studies the majority of patients were able to tolerate at least half the target dose. Mean doses in these trials were carvedilol 45mg, bisoprolol 6.6mg and metoprolol 159mg.

Calcium channel blockers

Calcium antagonists are effective antihypertensive agents but they may worsen heart failure. Short acting nifedipine, felodipine and diltiazem are best avoided in heart failure patients. If a calcium channel blocker is required (e.g. if there is co-existent angina) amlodipine is the drug of choice. This once daily preparation has no adverse effect on mortality or morbidity in patients with heart failure.

Angiotensin II receptor blockers (ARBs)

ARBs are a new class of drug with similar antihypertensive efficacy to ACE inhibitors. They block the action of angiotensin II at its receptor (similar to the action of ß-blockers at beta adrenoceptors). They are often combined with thiazide diuretics and are emerging as the best drugs for hypertensives with LVH (see Chapters on LVH and Hypertension in the Elderly).

ARB's have a superior side effect profile than ACE inhibitors but theoretical advantages over ACE inhibitors have not yet been proven in heart failure patients. The effect of ARB's on mortality in heart failure patients is still under investigation, with huge trials underway. The ELITE-II study demonstrated equivalence of losartan to captopril and ACE inhibitors remain the first choice for CHF patients[10]. ARB's should be considered in patients with CHF who are intolerant of ACE inhibitors. Trials of ACE inhibitor/ARB combinations are currently underway. As applies with ACE-inhibitors, acute renal failure can occur during intercurrent illness and patients should be advised.

Vasodilators

Although ACE inhibitors are the first choice antihypertensive in CHF, isosorbide dinitrate and hydralazine should be considered when ACE inhibitors are not tolerated. In combination, these two drugs have a modest beneficial effect on mortality and will improve symptoms. Isosorbide dinitrate should be commenced at a dose of 5-10mg tid increasing to 40mg tid. A ten-hour nitrate free period should be maintained to avoid nitrate tolerance. Hydralazine should be started at 10mg qid increasing gradually to 75mg qid.

Alpha Blockers

The doxazosin limb of the Antihypertensive and Lipid Lowering Treatment to Prevent Heart Attack Trial (ALLHAT) Study was recently discontinued due to an increasing trend towards congestive heart failure compared to the chlorthalidone group. Although the reason for this is unclear, doxazosin should probably be avoided in hypertensive patients with LV dysfunction.

Non-pharmacological measures

All patients with heart failure and hypertension should modify their lifestyle. Obesity, cigarette smoking and excess alcohol consumption must be reversed. Dietary advice should be reinforced. Reduced salt consumption and a low cholesterol diet are indicated. In particular, ACE inhibitors (and probably ARBs) are less effective in patients with a high salt diet, and are particularly potent when salt intake is restricted. Mild to moderate dynamic exercise such as walking or gentle bicycle riding should be encouraged. Isometric exercise such as weightlifting causes an acute increase in afterload stress to the LV and should be discouraged.

Summary

Hypertension is a significant risk factor for the development of congestive heart failure. Fortunately, a number of antihypertensives are also of proven benefit in the treatment of CHF. ACE inhibitors should be prescribed for all patients unless contraindicated. ß-blockers can reduce the risk of death in CHF patients but should be started cautiously in case worsening heart failure ensues. Angiotensin receptor antagonists or a combination of hydralazine and isosorbide dinitrate should be considered in patients intolerant of ACE inhibitors. Diuretics are of value in improving CHF symptoms. Calcium channel blockers may worsen heart failure with the exception of amlodipine. All patients should make appropriate lifestyle changes as an adjunct to drug therapy.

Key Points

- Hypertension is a major risk factor for the development of heart failure.

- ACE inhibitors should be prescribed unless absolutely contraindicated.

- ARBs may be alternative in ACE intolerant patients

- ACEIs and probably ARBs should be withheld during intercurrent illness or dehydration (risk of renal failure)

- Diuretics provide symptomatic benefit in congestive heart failure.
- ß-blockers can reduce mortality in CHF but should be initiated with caution.
- Spironolactone is valuable in low doses but great care must be taken to avoid hyperkalemia when used with ACE inhibitors or ARBs
- Lifestyle modifications are an essential adjunct to pharmacological therapy.

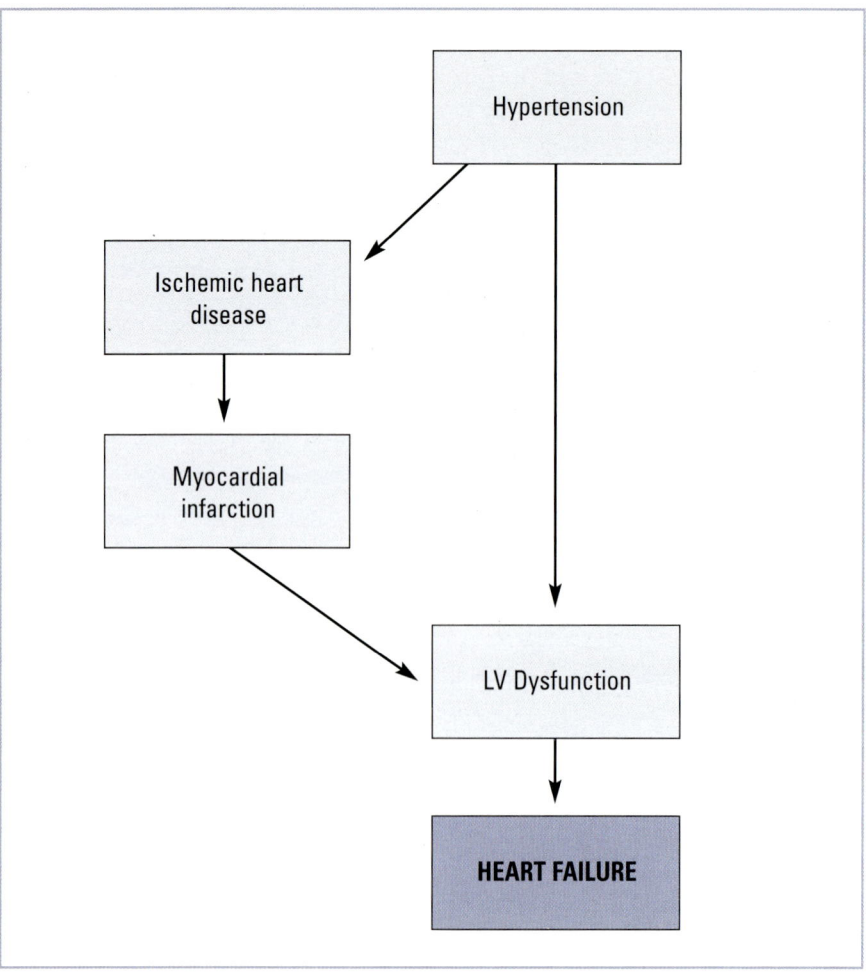

Figure 1. The link between hypertension and heart failure.

AGENT	SYMPTOMS	MORTALITY
ACE Inhibitor	Improved	Improved
ARB	Equivalent to ACEI	Equivalent to ACEI
Diuretic	Improved	Unknown
ß-blocker	Improve/worsen	Improved
Hydralazine/nitrate	Improved	Modest improvement
Calcium antagonists	May worsen	May worsen (Amlodipine safe)

Figure 4. Effects of antihypertensives in congestive heart failure.

References

1. Kannel WB, Belanger AJ: Epidemiology of heart failure. *Am Heart J* 1991;121:951-957.

2. SOLVD Investigators: Effect of enalapril on survival in patients with reduced left ventricular ejection fractions and congestive heart failure. *N Engl J Med* 1992;325:293-302.

3. Guidelines for the evaluation and management of heart failure. *Circulation* 1995;92:2764-2784.

4. Packer M, Poole-Wilson PA, Armstrong PW et al. Comparative effects of low and high doses of the angiotensin converting enzyme inhibitor, lisinopril, on morbidity and mortality in chronic heart failure. ATLAS Study Group. *Circulation* 1999;100:2312-8.

5. MERIT-HF Investigators. Effect of metoprolol CR/XL in chronic heart failure: metoprolol CR/XL randomised intervention trial in congestive heart failure. (MERIT-HF). *Lancet* 1999;353:2001-7. CIBIS

6. CIBIS-II Investigators. The cardiac insufficiency bisoprolol study II: a randomised trial. *Lancet* 1999;353:9-13.

7. Packer M, Bristow MR, Cohn JN et al. The effect of carvedilol on morbidity and mortality in patients with chronic heart failure. *N Engl J Med* 1996;334:1349-55.

8. Packer M, Coats AJS, Fowler MB et al. Effect of carvedilol on survival in severe chronic heart failure. *N Engl J Med* 2001;344:1651-8.

9. Dargie HJ. Effect of carvedilol on outcome after myocardial infarction in patients with left-ventricular dysfunction: the CAPRICORN randomised trial. *Lancet.* 357(9266):385-90, 2001 May 5.

10. Pitt B, Poole-Wilson P, Segal R et al. Effect of losartan compared with captopril on mortality in patients with symptomatic heart failure: randomised trial- the losartan heart failure survival study ELITE II. *Lancet* 2000;355:1582-87.

11. SHEP Cooperative Research Group: Prevention of stroke by antihypertensive drug treatment in older persons with isolated systolic hypertension. Final results of the Systolic Hypertension in the Elderly Program (SHEP). *JAMA* 1991;265:3255-3264.

CHAPTER 7

HYPERTENSION AND DIABETES MELLITUS *John Petrie*

Two million people are known to have diabetes in the UK with a further million thought to be undiagnosed. Similar figures may apply in other "westernized" societies. It has been recognized for over 20 years that type 2 diabetes and hypertension frequently co-exist (and may be pathophysiologically linked), but healthcare systems still tend to "compartmentalize" them. Thus, care of a person with a particular clinical profile can be delivered (according to various historical and/or geographical factors) in primary care, a "Hypertension" clinic, a "Diabetes" clinic, or a combination of the three (Figure 1).

People with type 2 diabetes have an average annual mortality of 5.4% - i.e. baseline "primary prevention" risk is equivalent to that usually seen in "secondary prevention".[1] The sheer numbers of cases of type 2 diabetes already diagnosed are such that consultant diabetologists may only be seeing 50% of known cases in their catchment's area and even then only on an annual basis. Diabetes clinics originally grew up around the concept of controlling blood glucose in people with type 1 diabetes using insulin.

Consultations may therefore focus disproportionately on blood glucose, while an elevated BP (if measured) may simply be communicated to the family doctor by letter with advice on monitoring/ treatment. This may even be seen as unwanted interference in "primary" prevention of CHD, which is regarded by some as the territory of "primary" care: action, if indeed it is required, may not be taken. Through their experience of this system, people with diabetes may themselves take home the idea that only blood glucose is important: "they can't be too worried about my blood pressure if my next appointment is in a year."

Before the era heralded by the UK Prospective Diabetes Study, significant cynicism existed concerning the possibilities of improving health outcomes in people with type 2 diabetes. However, the explosion of evidence over the last five years demonstrating large reductions in cardiovascular "endpoints" (i.e. myocardial infarction and stroke) with antihypertensive treatment in these subjects (Table 1) has resulted in a new therapeutic optimism.

A "glucocentric" approach is now recognized as anomalous and potentially counterproductive. There is a growing realization that modernization of present systems of care is required to implement evidence-based findings at a population level. Managed clinical networks are likely to be the best model to achieve this goal: comprehensive registers, efficient liaison between primary and secondary care, online data sharing and effective clinical audit. Examples of excellence already exist, but in many areas the situation is unsatisfactory and both leadership and resources are urgently required to turn the tide.

What are the benefits of treating hypertension in diabetes?

Evidence is now available from one large randomized controlled trial comparing "tight" and "less tight" BP-lowering strategies in people with diabetes (UKPDS) and also from various subgroup analyses of placebo-controlled trials of systolic ($\geq$160 mmHg) hypertension in which a large number of people with diabetes were included (Table 1). These have in general confirmed the statistical prediction that people with diabetes derive more absolute benefit from BP reduction than non-diabetic individuals (as a function of their elevated baseline risk).[2] Thus, in most trials, the relative risk reduction associated with a given treatment is translated into a higher absolute risk reduction when applied to subjects (with diabetes) in whom baseline cardiovascular risk is higher.

The UKPDS began investigating the effect of glycaemic control on outcomes in type 2 diabetes in 1977. After 10 years, the investigators realized that nearly 40% of the people recruited were hypertensive (i.e. had BP $\geq$ 160 and/ or $\geq$ 90 mmHg) or were already on antihypertensive treatment. Fortunately, they had the foresight to randomize these people into a BP-lowering study.

A "tight BP control" strategy based on atenolol and captopril (mean achieved BP 144/82 mmHg) vs. a "less tight" strategy (154/ 87 mmHg) ultimately resulted in a 44% reduction in stroke and a 32% reduction in a predefined endpoint of "deaths related to diabetes" (mainly accounted for by myocardial infarction and stroke). Other than the lack of a statistically significant reduction in myocardial infarction (when considered alone) in these middle-aged subjects, the findings were similar to the diabetes subgroup analysis of the chlorthalidone-based placebo-controlled Systolic Hypertension in the Elderly Program (SHEP) conducted in the US (published in 1996).

A further placebo-controlled trial conducted in Europe in elderly people - SYST-EUR – has also provided evidence that similar benefits are observed with a calcium channel blocker (CCB) based regime (albeit combined in 60% of cases with enalapril); in this trial, absolute and relative reductions in major endpoints were larger in the diabetes subgroup.

A surprising finding of UKPDS was that treatment of hypertension in people with diabetes was also associated with a reduction in *microvascular* (as well as macrovascular) endpoints, previously considered a result purely of hyperglycemia. In fact, the magnitude of reduction in these endpoints was similar to that noted in people allocated in the main study to intensive vs. conventional glucose control.

Diabetes Centre 1995	Hypertension Clinic 1995	Cardiovascular Prevention Clinic 2005
"I saw this 65-year-old man who has a five year history of type 2 diabetes mellitus today. HbA1c is good at 7.9 % on gliclazide 80mg daily. He has mild background retinopathy. We will see him for annual review in one year."	"I saw this 65-year-old man with essential hypertension today. He is tolerating therapy with atenolol 50mg and amlodipine 5mg daily. BP today was 150/95 mmHg (sitting), which is satisfactory. He has no LVH and electrolytes are normal. As you know, he has mild diabetes. We will see him in six months."	I saw this 65-year-old male non-smoker who has a five-year history of type 2 diabetes mellitus today. His blood pressure has settled to 140/ 90 mmHg on atenolol, amlodipine and ramipril. As it is not yet to "target" I have added in a thiazide diuretic. LDL cholesterol is 3.5 mmol/L and I have increased his simvastatin to 80mg daily. He is on 75mg aspirin daily. Glycosylated hemoglobin (DCCT aligned HbA1c) was satisfactory at 7.0% on gliclazide 80mg daily. BMI is 28 kg/m2 and I have prescribed an exercise programe. He has no background retinopathy or microalbuminuria.
Dr B.M. Stick P.S. His BP was 180/105 mmHg today - please recheck in your own surgery	Dr Sid O. Manometer P.S. His blood glucose was 12.3 mmol/L - please recheck in your own surgery	Dr E.A. Ming

Figure 1.

When to treat? - thresholds

As in non-diabetic subjects, detection of high BP is an opportunity to promote sensible measures such as weight reduction, salt restriction, exercise, increased fruit and vegetable intake and moderation of alcohol intake. The 1999 (third) revision of the

British Hypertension Society guidelines for the management of hypertension recommends that all people with diabetes and sustained BP elevated ≥140 mmHg systolic and/ or ≥90 mmHg diastolic over a period of weeks of non-pharmacological management should start antihypertensive treatment.[3] This recommendation was derived by calculating "numbers needed to treat" and is based on three assumptions: 1) baseline 10 year risk of CHD in people with diabetes is generally ≥ 15%; 2) antihypertensive therapy is associated with a relative risk reduction in CHD of 16% over a period of 10 years (cf. 38% for stroke, a less common outcome); and, 3) treating 40 people for five years is worthwhile to prevent one CHD event. This guidance predates the publication of MICRO-HOPE in which people with diabetes >55 years of age and one other risk factor and a mean baseline BP close to recommended target (142/80 mmHg) randomized to an ACE inhibitor (ramipril) vs. placebo. The investigators reported significant improvements in cardiovascular outcomes associated with ramipril therapy which were attributed to ACE inhibition rather than BP reduction as they were greater than would have been predicted from the reported small reduction in BP. However, a subsequent paper in which 24 hour ambulatory BP was recorded, showing a large fall in blood pressure with ramipril in a subset of patients, challenges this interpretation.

How low to go? - targets

The Hypertension Optimal Treatment trial (HOT) is the only large trial specifically to have examined this question. One of the largest hypertension trials to date, it was set up to examine the issue of whether BP lowering could be taken too far – "the J shaped curve." People were allocated at random to three target BPs (≤80, ≤85, and ≤90 mmHg) using the calcium channel blocker felodipine initially with subsequent addition of an ACE inhibitor or a ß-blockers and, if necessary, a diuretic.

The randomization was stratified such that 500 people with diabetes were allocated to each group. At the end of the study, achieved mean diastolic BP was 81, 83 and 85 mmHg in the three groups respectively. Total and cardiovascular mortality were similar in these three groups, with no suggestion of a J-shaped curve. Those with diabetes appeared to derive benefit from BP lowering to 81 vs. 83 mmHg (e.g. cardiovascular mortality 3.7 vs. 11.2/ 1000 patient years – a 67% relative risk reduction).

The investigators concluded on an "intention-to-treat" basis that target BP should be 140/85 mmHg in non-diabetic subjects and 140/80 mmHg in those with diabetes. The exact relevance to clinical systolic BP targets of these data is tempered by use of a BP measuring device conceded elsewhere by the authors to underestimate this parameter by 6 mmHg. However, the randomized data from HOT are the best available at present and there is no good evidence to underpin the 1997 target recommendation of 130/85 mmHg set by the US Joint National Committee on Prevention, Evaluation and Treatment of High Blood Pressure (JNC VI).[4]

It has been argued that people with diabetes and microalbuminuria (30-300 mg/day i.e. undetectable by standard clinical "dipstick" methods), in whom risk of cardiovascular disease is doubled with respect to their normalbuminuric counterparts, should be targeted for tight BP control and intensive risk factor modification. JNC VI advocates a target of 120/75 mmHg, based on extrapolation from evidence in advanced nephropathy (protein excretion > 1g/day). A number of trials have suggested potential benefits of ARBs over other agents for these patients (see chapter 10)

However, as current evidence suggests that relative risk reduction from BP and other interventions is similar across the spectrum of people with diabetes - independent of microalbuminuria status - the main justification for such an approach is that absolute risk reduction is likely to be higher as a function of higher baseline risk. Thus, "sub-dipstick" proteinuria may serve mainly to "flag up" people for whom failure to implement current thresholds and targets of BP control is particularly inexcusable.

Are newer agents better? Are calcium channel blockers dangerous?

Six major classes of antihypertensive agents exist: diuretics, b-blockers, calcium channel blockers, ACE inhibitors, angiotensin II type 1 receptor blockers and Alpha(α)-blockers "Centrally acting" agents are also available. As we have seen, clinical trials involving randomization of thousands of people were required to demonstrate the benefits of antihypertensive therapy in diabetes. Prior to the publication of these trials (SHEP, UKPDS, SYST-EUR), there was concern that the metabolic "adverse effects" of some antihypertensive agents (particularly diuretics and ß-blockers) might outweigh – or at least offset – the benefits. Many authors highlighted potentially deleterious effects of thiazide diuretics on surrogate end-points such as serum triglyceride concentrations, potassium levels and insulin sensitivity, preferring newer (more expensive) agents with "favorable" metabolic profiles.

Others pointed to evidence (lacking for other agents) that thiazides reduced rates of cardiovascular endpoints - even if some trials had excluded people with diabetes; according to this view, older "proven" agents were to be preferred until outcome based evidence emerged to support the use ACE inhibitors and calcium channel blockers.

UKPDS 39, in which captopril and atenolol were compared within the "tight" BP control group, showed similar event rates for major endpoints with both drugs. However, this by no means resolved debate as the statistical power provided by comparing 400 vs. 358 people fell far short of that required to exclude clinically relevant differences. Further heat - and very little light - was added with the publication of the Appropriate Blood Pressure Control in Diabetes study (ABCD) and the Fosinopril versus Amlodipine Cardiovascular Events study (FACET).

Both trials were small and set up to examine aspects of diabetes care other than cardiovascular endpoints, for which they had insufficient power. Their message was that calcium channel blockers might be inferior to ACE inhibitors in people with diabetes, and possibly dangerous. Given the results of later trials involving tens of thousands of people, this may well have been a result of type 1 statistical error.

The Captopril Prevention Project (CAPPP), the Swedish Trial in Older Patients 2 (STOP-2), the Nordic Diltiazem study (NORDIL) and the International Nifedipine GITS study (INSIGHT) all recruited a significant proportion of patients with diabetes and contributed to this increasingly complex debate (Table 1). All were open with blinded endpoints and evaluated the effects of two (or three) BP lowering strategies on cardiovascular endpoints. All were careful to prespecify both single and composite endpoints of interest in order to avoid the temptation *post hoc* to emphasize findings which might show artefactual "statistically significant" differences as a result of multiple comparisons. Randomisation problems were detectable in some centers contributing to the published results of CAPPP. In INSIGHT, nine centers were excluded from the final analyses after independent monitoring cast doubt on the existence of some subjects.

Imperfections not withstanding, results from the above trials in general supported the notion that the agents in question had similar effects on endpoints strongly related to their ability to lower BP. However, some intriguing discrepancies have emerged with respect to specific endpoints. For example, in comparing INSIGHT and NORDIL, both of which compared calcium channel blockers with "older" agents, stroke risk was reduced by calcium channel blockers only in NORDIL; however, heart failure risk appeared to be increased only in INSIGHT.

In CAPPP, stroke risk appeared to be considerably elevated in non-diabetic subjects in the captopril arm. This was attributed by the investigators to higher BP at randomization and indeed was not observed in the subgroup of people with diabetes in whom baseline BP was similar. A new debate has thus been generated – are some agents more effective at preventing certain "cause-specific" outcomes (e.g. stroke vs. CHD vs. heart failure)? Should antihypertensive therapy therefore be tailored according to risk in individuals (perhaps determined from DNA analysis) or in populations (CHD risk higher in Western countries, stroke risk higher in Asian countries)?

Meta-analysis of these trials concluded that evidence for differences between outcomes based on different drug classes was weak. This conclusion has in general been supported by recently published data from the largest ever blood pressure study: Antihypertensive and Lipid Lowering Treatment to prevent Heart Attack Trial (ALLHAT).[6] 33,357 subjects (12063 with diabetes as a pre-specified subgroup) were randomized with the aim of comparing the effect on cardiovascular endpoints of three newer anti-hypertensive drug classes (amlodipine, lisinopril, doxazosin) with a diuretic (chlorthalidone) based regimen. After a mean follow-up of 4.9 years, there was no difference in the relative risk of the primary outcome (combined fatal CHD or non-fatal myocardial infarction) or in all-cause mortality between amlodipine, doxazosin and the diuretic. Overall, results appeared very similar for patients with and without diabetes, although few data on adverse events were reported in the initial paper (December 2002). It should be noted that the doxazosin arm was discontinued early in 2000 because of an excess of heart failure events with respect to diuretic therapy, although doxazosin is rarely used as monotherapy in clinical practice.

One clinical scenario in which there may be a genuine difference between drug classes is for patients with left ventricular hypertrophy (LVH). The Losartan Intervention For Endpoint reduction (LIFE) study randomized over 9000 hypertensive subjects with LVH (1195 with diabetes) to losartan or atenolol.[7] Remarkably, losartan reduced sudden cardiac death by 40% compared to atenolol, a drug favored by cardiologists as protective against sudden cardiac death. There was a 37% reduction (unadjusted hazard ratio 0.57-0.95, p=0.017) in the relative risk of the primary composite endpoint (cardiovascular mortality, stroke and myocardial infarction) in the diabetics subgroup, but there was no significant difference in the relative risk of the single end-points of myocardial infarction or stroke. The findings of LIFE have not at the time of writing been integrated into diabetes care, and many "annual review" diabetic clinic protocols do not yet include the recording of an ECG.

In real life, a high proportion of people with diabetes require three or more agents (a third at eight years in UKPDS) to achieve adequate control, while co-morbidity, contra-indications and unwanted effects usually narrow the range of options available for a particular individual. However, polypharmacy is less appropriate for those in the UK who do not qualify for exemption from prescription charges (i.e. those not requiring oral hypoglycemic agents or insulin) and is likely to affect concordance with therapy.

A multi-faceted approach to primary prevention
While we have emphasized BP control in diabetes, it has been calculated that smoking cessation is the single intervention likely to produce most benefit in terms of outcome in those patients eligible. It is regrettable that to date there have been few intervention studies specifically in people with diabetes, who have higher smoking rates (>30%) than seen in the general population. Although absolute rates of quitting at six months may appear low at first sight (nicotine patches 12% vs. placebo 8% in non-diabetic subjects), worthwhile benefits are likely to result from this 50% relative increase in smoking cessation in a population at high baseline risk of cardiovascular disease.

Aspirin was clearly associated with decreased myocardial infarction (but not stroke) in the HOT trial although it was associated with a nearly doubling in rates of severe bleeding (1.3 vs 0.7%). Current recommendations are that it should be used in all hypertensive people with a 10 year CHD risk of ≥15%[3] or ≥30%[5] as calculated using to the Joint British Societies Coronary Risk Prediction Chart (see British National Formulary) provided a contraindication is not present; in practice this should include most middle-aged adults with diabetes.

Current recommendations on statin therapy for primary prevention of cardiovascular disease in people with diabetes are very much in evolution following the publication of the Heart Protection Study,[8] but increasingly will follow the Atherosclerosis Treatment and Prevention III guideline of the U.S. National Heart, Lung and Blood Institute in considering diabetes as a "CHD risk equivalent." Thus, in terms of cholesterol lowering, adults with diabetes will be treated "as if" they already have overt coronary heart disease, with correspondingly lower thresholds and targets, and perhaps even "statins for all."

Implementation
For those people who are known to have both hypertension and diabetes, and who are inclined to take prescribed medication, controlling BP with the available agents is usually relatively simple; resistant hypertension is an indication for further investigation. As already implied, the greater challenge is to implement optimal and equitable health care (as represented by current evidence) for all people in the population with initially asymptomatic but ultimately serious chronic conditions such as hypertension and diabetes. The key steps in this process are likely to be establishment of accurate registers, appointment of more community-based diabetes specialist nurses, improving communication between "primary" and "secondary" care, information management and technology, re-education of health professionals, and education/empowerment of people with diabetes.

Conclusions
A substantial body of evidence now suggests that attempts to lower BP are at least as effective as efforts to improve glycemic control in terms of preventing large and small vessel complications of diabetes. Thus, the burden of excess cardiovascular morbidity and mortality associated with type 2 diabetes may not be inevitable. On theoretical grounds, antihypertensive therapy should be initiated if either systolic BP is consistently greater than 140 mmHg or diastolic BP is consistently greater than 90 mmHg. The best target BP is uncertain but is around 140/80 mmHg for people with diabetes (on the basis of the HOT trial); combination therapy will often be required to achieve this.

Every consultation should be an opportunity to modify cardiovascular risk. Most people will need more than one drug to achieve BP targets, so obsessive debate regarding minor differences between drug classes is inappropriate. Further research is required into methods of implementing what is already known on a population-wide basis.

Key points

- Management of smoking, BP and lipids is just as important as controlling blood glucose in people with diabetes

- The absolute benefit of therapeutic interventions is higher in people with diabetes as a function of their elevated baseline risk

- BP lowering using diuretics, ß-blockers, calcium channel blockers, ACE inhibitors and angiotensin II receptor blockers (alone or in appropriate combinations) results in long term decreased risk of cardiovascular disease

- Strong evidence-based guidelines now exist, but implementation remains a challenge

References

*all major trials cited in the text are cited in full in:

Blood Pressure Lowering Treatment Trialists' Collaboration. Effects of ACE inhibitors, calcium antagonists, and other blood pressure-lowering drugs on mortality and major cardiovascular morbidity. *Lancet* 2000; 356: 1955-1964.

1) Donnelly, R., Emslie-Smith,A.M., Gardner, I.D., Morris, A.D. Vascular complications of diabetes. *Br Med J* 2000; 320: 1062-1066.

2) Yudkin JS. How can we best prolong life? Benefits of coronary risk factor reduction in non-diabetic and diabetic subjects. *Br Med J* 1993; 306: 1313-1318.

3) Ramsay, L.E., Williams, B., Johnston, G.D. et al. Guidelines for the management of hypertension: report of the third working party of the British Hypertension Society. *J Hum Hypertens* 1999; 13: 569-592. (also www.hyp.ac.uk/bhsinfo/1000917.pdf)

4) The Sixth Report of the Joint National Committee on Prevention, Evaluation, Detection and Treatment of High Blood Pressure. *Arch Intern Med* 1997; 157: 2413-2446.

5) Scottish Intercollegiate Guidelines Network 40. Lipids and the Primary Prevention of CHD. Edinburgh: *Royal College of Physicians*, 1999.

6) ALLHAT Collaborative Group. Major outcomes in high-risk hypertensive patients randomized to ACE inhibitor or calcium channel blocker vs diuretic: the Antihypertensive and Lipid Lowering Treatment to prevent Heart Attack Trial (ALLHAT). *JAMA* 2002;287:2981-2997

7) Lindholm LH, Ibsen H, Dahlof B et al. Cardiovascular morbidity and mortality in patients with diabetes in the Losartan Intervention For Endpoint reduction in hypertension study (LIFE): a randomised trial against atenolol. *Lancet* 2002; 359: 1004-1010.

8) Heart Protection Study Collaborative Group. MRC/BHF Heart Protection study of cholesterol lowering with simvastatin in 20 536 high-risk individuals: a randomised placebo-controlled trial. *Lancet* 2002; 360:7-22.

Study (year)	*n* randomized	*n* diabetes	% female	mean age	Main comparison	Odds Ratio MI (p value)φ	Odds ratio Stroke (p value)φ	Comments
SHEP (1991)	4736	583	58	71	Chlorthalidone vs. placebo	0.77 (0.57-1.05)	0.62 (0.46-0.83)	
SHEP Diabetes (1996)		583	50	70	Chlorthalidone vs. placebo	0.46 (0.24-0.88)	0.78 (0.45-1.34)	
SYST-EUR (1997)	4695	492	66.8	70	Nitrendipine vs. placebo	0.78 (0.10)	0.64 (0.02)	
		492			Nitrendipine vs. placebo	0.43 (0.06)	0.31 (0.02)	
UKPDS 38 (1998)	1148	1148	44	56	Tight (144/82mmHg) vs. less tight (154/87 mmHg)	0.79 (0.13)	0.56 (0.013)	Microvascular complications also reduced
UKPDS 39 (1998)	758	758	46	56	Captopril vs. atenolol	1.20 (0.35)	1.12 (0.74)	
ABCD (1998)	470	470	33	57	Nisoldipine vs enalapril	5.5 (2.1-14.6)	1.6 (0.6-4.2)	CHD and stroke outcomes were secondary endpoints and total number of events was small
FACET (1998)	380	380	40	63	Amlodipine v fosinopril	1.29 (>0.1)	2.56 (>0.1)	Headline combined (secondary) end point "any major cardiovascular event" significantly higher in calcium anatagonist group – see text
HOT (1998)	18790	1501	47	61.5	Target diastolic BPs: <80 vs. <85 vs <90 mmHg	0.73 (0.05)	0.95 (0.74)	
		1501	not stated	not stated	Target diastolic BPs: <80 vs. <85 vs <90 mmHg (diabetes subgroup)	0.49 (0.11)	0.70 (0.34)	
STOP-2 (1999)	6614	719	66.8	76	ACE I vs. conventional	0.90 (0.80)	0.90 (0.24)	Headline lower incidence of MI in ACE I group should be interpreted with caution as 48 statistical comparisons were made. 10-11% patients allocated to each treatment regime had diabetes.
					ACE I vs. CCB	0.77 (0.016)	1.02 (0.64)	
					CCB vs. conventional	1.10 (0.13)	0.66 (0.16)	
CAPPP (1999)	10985	572	52	46	Captopril vs. conventional	0.94 (0.30)	1.25 (0.04)	
		572			Captopril vs. conventional (diabetic subgroup)	0.67 (0.03)	1.02 (0.95)	
INSIGHT (2000)	6321	1302	54	65	Nifedipine GITS vs. co-amilozide	1.11 (0.34)	1.11 (0.34)	Full diabetes subgroup analysis not presented to date
NORDIL (2000)	10881	727	51	60	Diltiazem vs. diuretic/ ß-blocker	0.80 (0.04)	1.16 (0.17)	
MICRO-HOPE (2000)	3577	3577	65	37	Ramipril v placebo	0.78 (0.01)	0.67 (0.007)	
ALLHAT (2000)	24335	8633	47	67	Doxazosin v Chlorthalidone	1.10 (0.05)	1.19 (0.04)	Discontinued early due to excess events (congestive heart failure) with respect to diuretics.

Study (year)	*n* randomized	*n* diabetes	% female	mean age	Main comparison	Odds Ratio MI (p value)ϕ	Odds ratio Stroke (p value)ϕ	Comments
ALLHAT diabetes (2002)[6]	33357	12063	47	67	Amlodipine v Chlorthalidone	0.99 (0.87-1.13)	0.90 (0.75-1.08)	
ALLHAT diabetes (2002)[6]	33357 9193	12063 1195 1195	47 54 53	67 67 67	Lisinopril v Chlorthalidone	1.00 (0.87-1.14)	1.07 (0.90-1.28)	
LIFE (2002)[7]					Losartan v atenolol	1.05 (0.628)	0.74 (0.0006)	
					Losartan v atenolol	0.81 (0.318)	0.78 (0.190)	Subjects with LVH-37% reduction in composite cardiovascular mortality for losartan compared with atenolol (p=0.028)

Table 1.　　　　　　　　　　　ϕ *Values in brackets are p values or 95% confidence intervals*
CCB = calcium channel blocker

CHAPTER 8

HYPERTENSION IN OLDER PATIENTS
Jacqueline Taylor and Adrian Brady

Introduction

A major non-fatal stroke is arguably the worst medical disaster that can happen to a patient. No one is at greater risk than the elderly hypertensive.

The prevalence of hypertension rises with age and depending on the threshold used 25%-50% of patients over the age of 65 are hypertensive. Indeed, applying the modern definition of high blood pressure as >140/90 mm Hg, the 2000 Health Survey of England, which screened a random population sample of 2024 individuals over 65 shows that *almost 80% of the elderly* have uncontrolled blood pressure[11].

Systolic blood pressure relates more closely to vascular complications than diastolic blood pressure and systolic hypertension is particularly common in this age group. Blood pressure is the single most modifiable risk factor for diseases, which carry a high mortality and great burden of disability such as myocardial infarction, stroke and congestive heart failure. In addition, other cardiovascular risk factors particularly diabetes, hyperlipidemia, left ventricular hypertrophy and obesity are more common in older patients than in middle-aged patients with hypertension.

As such, older patients with hypertension have a higher risk of cardiovascular mortality and morbidity than their younger counterparts. Despite this there remains reluctance amongst some doctors to adequately treat hypertension in older patients. Undoubtedly their cormorbidities and the subsequent potential for drug interactions and adverse effects can make them a complex group to treat. However, in absolute terms they have the most to gain from good blood pressure control and with careful management and individualized treatment this can be achieved.

Most elderly hypertensives develop systolic hypertension, with normal diastolic levels. The pathophysiology of isolated systolic hypertension (ISH) is different to the essential hypertension of middle age. Ageing increases the stiffness of the aorta and large conducting vessels. Ejection of blood into the aorta causes a more rapid rise in pressure because of reduced compliance of these large vessels. There is an increase in pulse wave velocity which has an additional effect. Furthermore there is increased peripheral resistance as the resistance arteries stiffen up with age. The aortic systolic pulse wave bounces off this stiff vascular resistance wall and accentuates the high systolic level (Figure 1).

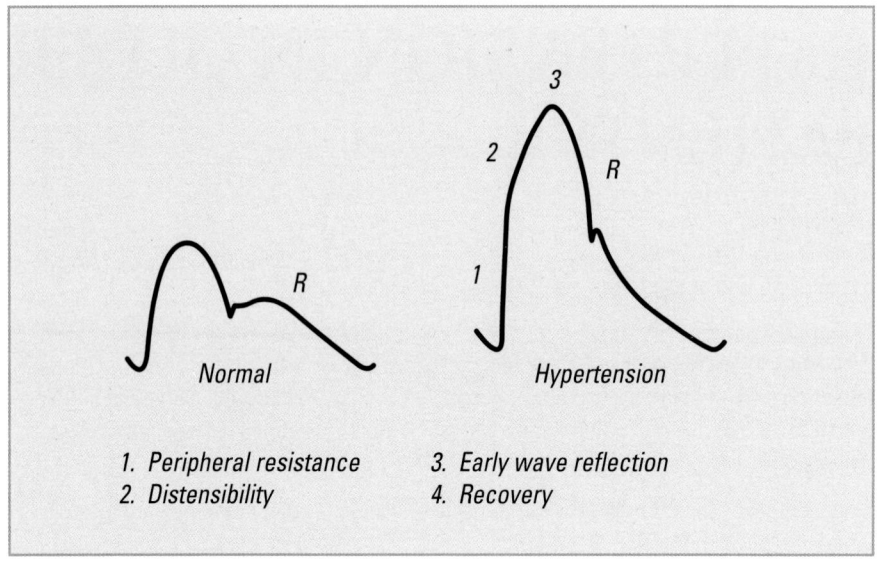

Figure 1. Aortic pressure waves in ISH.

What Is The Evidence That Treatment Of Hypertension Over The Age Of 65 Is Of Benefit?

Since 1985 a number of landmark studies have been published which have shown the value of treating both combined systolic/diastolic hypertension and isolated systolic hypertension in older patients. Overall the treatment effect on stroke has been more favorable than on cardiovascular events: Meta-analysis of randomized controlled trials suggest a 30%-40% reduction of morbidity and mortality from stroke and a 20-25% reduction in coronary heart disease events and mortality.

Given that the prevalence of cardiovascular risk factors was lower among trial patients than the general population of elderly hypertensives, the absolute benefits are likely to be even greater. There is, therefore, evidence that at least up to the age of 80-85 years that treatment is beneficial. The picture in the over 85s is less clear, but the HYVET Study, which is ongoing (Treatment of Hypertension in the Very Elderly) will hopefully show whether or not the very elderly receive the same benefits of treatment. Early results from HYVET show better morbidity but no improvement in mortality at one year (C Bulpitt, presented at the European Society of Hypertension, Prague, June 2002).

How Far Should Blood Pressure Be Lowered?

It is clearly important that treatment of an asymptomatic condition does not result in symptomatic postural hypotension and subsequent falls, and concerns about these potential problems have resulted in an over-conservative approach to blood pressure lowering. Until recently there has been little guidance as to what target blood pressure should be.

The HOT Study, however, has provided some answers[1]. This study of 18,790 patients, mean age 61.5 (range 50-80) randomly assigned patients to a target diastolic blood pressure of <90, <85 or <80 mmHg. Treatment was with a calcium channel blocker with the addition of ACE Inhibitor, ß-Blocker or diuretic if required to reach target blood pressure. The study showed that blood pressure could be safely lowered to 140/90 but that overall further reduction did not confer any mortality or morbidity advantage. Only in the sub-population of diabetic patients did aggressive lowering of blood pressure result in any further statistical reduction of major cardiovascular events. It does, therefore, seem reasonable to aim for a target blood pressure of 140/90.

The belief by some authors in a J shaped relationship between mortality and diastolic blood pressure has hindered the treatment of hypertension in the elderly. While frail ill patients may have low blood pressure, there is no evidence that aggressive BP lowering is bad for you. The opposite is true, and modern BP targets are much tougher than they were, since all the evidence points to worthwhile reductions in stroke and MI when such targets are reached. We should probably stop lowering systolic blood pressure if the diastolic level falls below < 55 mm Hg. However, this still leaves plenty of opportunity to work hard for our patients to achieve aggressive systolic BP lowering.

How Should Hypertension Be Treated?

Patients with diastolic blood pressure >=90 mmHg. or systolic blood pressure >=160 mmHg, which is persistent, i.e. measured on three separate occasions, should be considered for treatment of hypertension. However, not all patients who are considered for treatment should receive it. For example, a frail 90-year-old woman with recurrent falls and advanced malignancy is unlikely to benefit significantly from treatment of hypertension. Decisions must be made on an individual basis taking the patient's cormorbidities into account. However, it must be reiterated that in the vast majority of cases the potential benefits of treatment of hypertension are considerable.

1. Non-Pharmacological Treatment

Changes in lifestyle are harder to achieve in older patients. However, non-pharmacological measures play an important part in treating blood pressure and may obviate the need for drugs. Patients should be advised on weight reduction, the avoidance of excessive alcohol intake, reduction in salt intake and regular physical activity. Non-steroidal anti-inflammetory drugs should be avoided if possible. ACE inhibitor therapy is particularly sensitive to salt intake, and ACEIs work best with a degree of sodium restriction.

2. Modification of Cardiovascular Risk Factors

Hypertension is one of many cardiovascular risk factors that an individual may carry. The presence of other risk factors may well influence the threshold at which hypertension is treated. In addition to the lifestyle measures mentioned above, patients should be advised to stop smoking and to reduce saturated fat intake.

There is good evidence from the 4S, Care, LIPID and most importantly the Heart Protection Study (see chapter on Hypertension, Hyperlipidemia and estimation of cardiovascular risk) that cholesterol lowering in patients with ischemic heart disease at least up to the age of 80 reduces the number of ischemic vascular events including stroke. Further new evidence from the Heart Protection Study strengthens arguments to treat high cholesterol in any individual with risk factors for cardiovascular disease, almost regardless of the cholesterol level – lower is always better.

3. Drug Treatment

In general terms, drug treatment should be instituted at small doses gradually titrated upwards and patients carefully monitored for postural hypotension and other adverse effects. Older patients often have other cormorbidities which necessitate drug treatment. They may well have functional impairments, and selection of anti-hypertensive drugs must therefore be tailored to the individual. There is a large body of evidence from landmark studies on the efficacy of Thiazide diuretics, ß-Blockers and calcium channel blockers:

(a) Thiazide Diuretics

Thiazide Diuretics are inexpensive and effective. This was shown in the landmark SHEP and MRC trials in the early 1990s [2,3]. Higher doses confer no benefit and result in a greater incidence of adverse effects, in particular, electrolyte disturbance. They may precipitate or aggravate urinary incontinence, and gout. These problems coupled with concerns over their long term adverse metabolic effects have resulted in a decline in their use. However, postural hypotension is not common and we use them as first line agents. The recent ALLHAT trial [10] confirms their position as first line therapy for uncomplicated patients.

(b) ß-Blockers

ß-Blockers have proven efficacy as anti-hypertensive agents. However, older patients are more likely to have a contra-indication to treatment with ß-Blockers, such as peripheral vascular disease or chronic obstructive airways disease. They are drugs of choice in patients with co-existent angina and there is now a large body of evidence (albeit in younger patients) that they reduce morbidity and mortality in heart failure. They may be less effective in systolic hypertension, and are not now generally recommended as first-line agents in older patients.

(c) Calcium Channel Blocking Agents

There is good evidence from SystEur, HOT[4,1] and other trials that long acting preparations are safe and effective anti-hypertensive agents. As a group they can cause headache, flushing and reflex tachycardia, but ankle edema and constipation are the most troublesome adverse effects in older patients. Contra-indications to treatment vary with individual agents. Verapamil is a negative inotrope and slows A.V. conduction. There is a suggestion however that it improves diastolic function. Amlodipine may be safer than other CCBs in patients with congestive heart failure. We use long acting dihydropyridine CCBs as alternative first or first add-on therapy besides thiazide diuretics.

(d) ACE Inhibitors

The CAPPP study[5] and the STOP-2[6] studies looked at the long term effect of ACE Inhibitor treatment of hypertension, although an ACE Inhibitor was add-on treatment in SystEur and the HOT study. However, there is a very large body of evidence, at least in the young elderly, that ACE Inhibitors reduce mortality and morbidity in the treatment of congestive heart failure.

As such, ACE Inhibitors are probably agents of choice in patients who have both hypertension and congestive heart failure. Older patients have a high incidence of occult reno-vascular disease and careful monitoring of renal function is required before initiation and during upwards titration of an ACE Inhibitor. Moreover, older patients may develop impairment of renal function long after they have been stabilized on an ACE Inhibitor if they become volume depleted or develop inter-current illness. A low threshold for checking renal function is essential in managing these patients. The ACE inhibitor, perindopril, when combined with a thiazide, has been shown to have efficacy in prevention of stroke and cardiac events in patients with overt cerebrovascular disease (see chapter on HT and Stroke).

(e) Angiotensin receptor antagonists (ARBs)

ARBs Angiotensin blockers produce comparable reductions in blood pressure to other anti-hypertensive agents. Losartan has recently been shown in the recent, large LIFE trial [7] to have a substantially better outcome than atenolol-based therapy in patients with LVH for near identical blood pressure lowering. Indeed, among patients with ISH treated with Losartan the results were remarkably superior to atenolol based therapy, suggesting that therapy based on ARBs may have particular advantages for some patients (Figures 2 and 3). Results in the LIFE trial were especially favorable among diabetics and in patients with systolic hypertension [8].

Another ARB, candesartan has also been shown in 2002 in the SCOPE trial [9] to have an important benefit over existing conventional antihypertensive therapy in the reduction of risk of stroke in elderly hypertensives. ARBs will become increasingly widely used for elderly hypertensives, especially if they have LVH or diabetes.

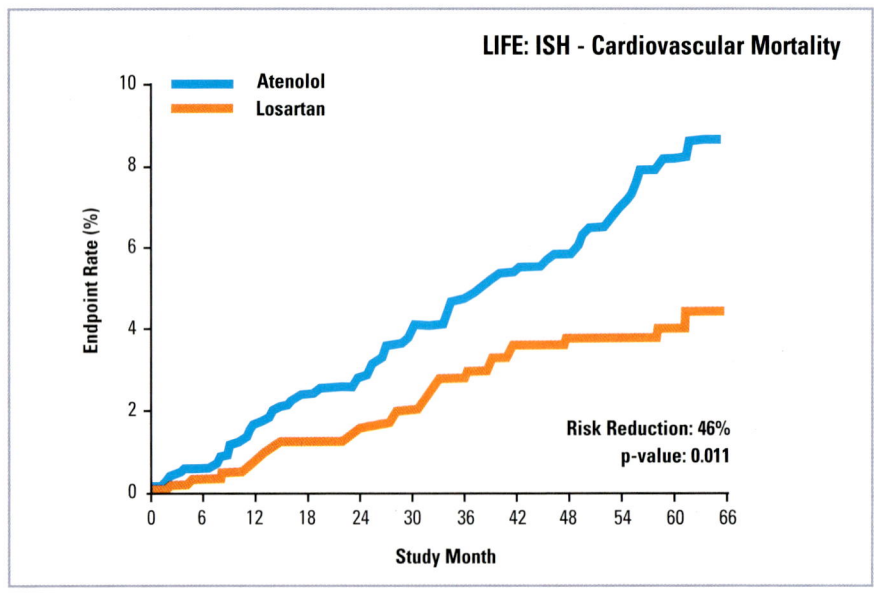

Figure 2. Effect of the ARB Losartan on cardiovascular mortality in elderly patients with hypertension, LVH and isolated systolic HT [8].

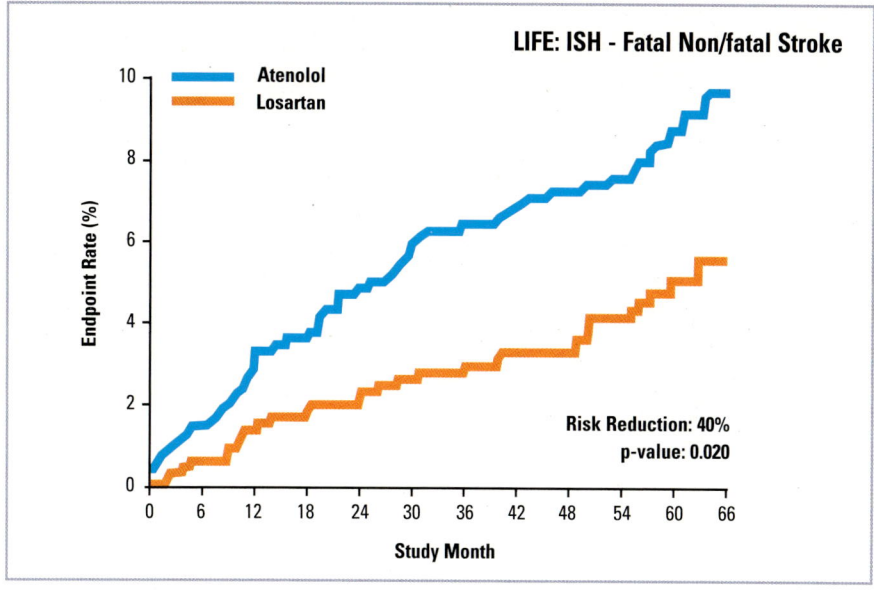

Figure 3. Effect of losartan on stroke in elderly patients with hypertension, LVH and isolated systolic HT[8].

Conclusions

Hypertension is very common in older patients. Indeed, most elderly individuals are hypertensive. There is clear evidence that lowering blood pressure reduces cardiovascular events. Treatment decision must be made on an individual basis and target blood pressure should probably be 140/90 mm Hg. By effectively treating hypertension we have the opportunity to reduce the incidence of diseases which cause significant mortality but more importantly morbidity and disability in older patients.

- Preventing stroke is the most important intervention we can make

- Systolic hypertension is the commonest type of hypertension in the elderly

- Thiazides, the long acting calcium channel blockers nifedipine, once daily modified release preparation and amlodipine, and the ARBs losartan (and candesartan to be published) have the most supportive evidence.

References

1. Hansson L, et al. The hypertension optimal treatment study. *Lancet* 1998;351:1755

2. SHEP Cooperative Research Group. SHEP trial. *JAMA* 1991;265:3255-64.

3. MRC working party. Treatment of mild hypertension in the elderly. *Br Med J* 1992;304:405.

4. Staessen JA, et al. Morbidity and mortality in the Syst-Eur trial. *Lancet* 1997;350:757-64.

5. L Hansson et al. The CAPPP trial. *Lancet* 1999;353:611-16.

6. Hansson L, et al. (STOP 2). *Lancet* 1999; 354: 1751-56

7. Kjeldsen SE, Dahlof B, Devereux, et al. Effects of Losartan on Cardiovascular morbidity and mortality in patients with isolated systolic hypertension and left ventricular hypertrophy. *JAMA* 2002;288:1491-1498.

8. Dahlof B, Devereux RB, et al. Cardiovascular morbidity and mortality in the Losartan for Endpoint reduction in hypertension study. *Lancet* 2002;359:995-1003

9. SCOPE trial L Hansson, et al. European Society of Hypertension, *Prague* 2002

10. ALLHAT Collaborative Group. Major outcomes in high-risk hypertensive patients randomised to ACE inhibitor or calcium channel blocker vs diuretic: the Antihypertensive and Lipid Lowering Treatment to prevent Heart Attack Trial (ALLHAT). *JAMA* 2002;287:2981-2997.

11. Primatesta P and Poulter NR, Br Soc HT, Cambridge, Sept 02.

CHAPTER 9

HYPERTENSION IN CHILDREN AND YOUNG ADULTS
Andrew Clark and Adrian Brady

Hypertension is less common in children than in adults, and where it occurs, is more likely to have an underlying cause. Nevertheless, essential hypertension is still the commonest cause of hypertension in the young.

Normal ranges
Normal ranges for blood pressure in children are published.[1] Blood pressure is normally distributed, and so hypertension is diagnosed in relation to the normal distribution. In general, a diastolic pressure above 85 mmHg under the age of 12 years, and above 90 over the age of 12 is abnormal. It is important to measure blood pressure with an appropriately sized blood pressure cuff in the young. A large cuff will give a spuriously lower blood pressure, and a small cuff an elevated pressure.

Causes of hypertension
The finding of hypertension in a child should prompt a search for possible primary causes (see table 1). The older the child, the more likely that hypertension is essential.

Coarctation of the aorta
Coarctation is a congenital cardiovascular defect where the isthmus of the aorta (the segment of the arch between the left subclavian artery and the insertion of the ductus arteriosus) fails to develop properly. The result is a shelf projecting into the aortic lumen from the posterolateral wall of the aorta. Other cardiac anomalies, particularly bicuspid aortic valve, are commonly associated with coarctation. Turner's syndrome is associated with coarctation.

Blood supply to the lower body is then principally via collateral vessels, mainly the internal mammary (thoracic) and intercostal arteries. Upper body hypertension arises from the decrease in renal perfusion.

Presentation. A severe coarctation presents early with heart failure in the neonate. However, the majority of patients is asymptomatic, and is picked up on routine surveillance by the presence of radiofemoral delay. It is thus not surprising that many cases of coarctation go unrecognized into adolescence and adult life. Occasional patients complain of headaches, and even more rarely of claudication. Most patients present as incidentally noticed hypertension.

Examination. Blood pressure is elevated in the arms, or just the right arm if the coarct is proximal to the left subclavian artery, and is low, or even unrecordable, in the legs. The femoral pulses may be impalpable, but there is usually radio-femoral delay, that is a delay between the pulse felt at the radial artery and the femoral. The lesion itself may give rise to a systolic murmur. There may be a continuous murmur from the collaterals, usually heard best over the back. Retinal changes are less commonly seen than with other forms of hypertension.

Investigations. The ECG shows left ventricular hypertrophy. Chest X ray demonstrates rib notching due to the enlarged collaterals. The ascending aorta is dilated, as is the descending aorta beyond the coarctation, giving rise to the so-called "3" sign. Echocardiography will visualize the coarctation, and allow estimation of the pressure drop across it. Associated defects, particularly bicuspid aortic valve, can be identified. Echocardiographic windows are less reliable with increasing age of the patient.

Cardiac catheterization demonstrates the defect, the gradient across it and any associated abnormalities. Particularly important for the surgeon is knowledge of the origin of the subclavian vessels. Anomalous origin from the distal aorta can cause difficulties at operation.

Natural history. Coarctation is compatible will long term survival, but unoperated, approximately 50% of patients will be dead by the age of 30. Problems are of cerebral hemorrhage from associated Berry aneurysms, aortic rupture. Endocarditis occurs on the bicuspid aortic valve, and endarteritis less commonly at the coarctation site. Left ventricular failure may occur, but is rare before the age of 40.

Treatment. Coarctation needs surgical treatment at whatever age it is discovered. Older repair techniques included excision of the abnormal segment with a patch repair or an end-to-end anastamosis, or an interposition graft. The modern approach is a flap repair, using the left subclavian artery as the patch to widen the coarctation site.

Surgical repair can be complicated by paraplegia due to damage to the anterior spinal arteries. Balloon dilation of the coarctation may avoid this problem, but remains controversial as a primary repair. The ballooned site can be stented.

Follow-up. All patients with coarctation repair should be followed up long term. Hypertension commonly persists after repair. Exercise induced hypertension is particularly marked. Hypertension should be treated vigorously.

Problems with repair itself include aneurysm formation and rupture. Follow-up should include regular imaging of the repair site, particularly in those with a patch repair. Re-coarctation may occur, and can be treated with angioplasty and stent insertion.

Renal artery stenosis

In younger patients, renal artery stenosis (RAS) is due to fibromuscular hyperplasia within the artery wall rather than atherosclerosis. It affects young women more often than men. In about a quarter of cases, it is bilateral. There is usually a single, discrete lesion in the main renal artery, although the branches my be involved.

Presentation. Hypertension associated with RAS is often severe, or accelerated, and may be of abrupt onset. It often proves resistant to standard therapy, and is first suspected when a patient fails to respond to combination therapy. Occasionally a patient might present with heart failure. An important clue is abrupt worsening of renal function when starting treatment with an ACE inhibitor. The only clue on physical examination may be an abdominal bruit, but this is by no means always heard in RAS.

Investigations. There may be elevation of creatinine, especially where RAS is bilateral. Ultrasound may reveal asymmetry of kidney size. Isotopic renography after captopril challenge may be helpful. In the kidney with RAS, captopril produces acute ischemia, and the renogram will show unequal excretion. Intravenous pyelography is no longer recommended.

Renal artery ultrasound with Doppler measurements of blood flow is proving helpful in experienced hands. Magnetic resonance angiography may become more widely available and will replace what was previously the definitive investigation, renal arteriography. These two test both delineate the anatomy of both renal arteries accurately and demonstrate any intra-renal arterial pathology.

Treatment. Treating the RAS itself relieves the hypertension in many patients. Although some continue to be hypertensive, the blood pressure is much easier to control. Angioplasty and stenting of the renal arteries is now possible, and easier for the patient than open operation.

Mineralocorticoid syndromes

The description of rare metabolic syndromes of hypertension has generated interest for the possible light they might shed on essential hypertension. The principle mineralocorticoid, aldosterone, causes sodium retention in the distal convoluted tubule in exchange for potassium. Hyperalosteronism (Conn's syndrome) is a rare cause of hypertension characterized by hypokalemia and a low plasma renin activity (renin is suppressed by the raised aldosterone).

Cortisol is a potent mineralocorticoid. It is normally prevented from exerting its effects by being converted to cortisone in the kidney by 11ß hydroxysteroid dehydrogenase

(11ßHSD). In the syndrome of apparent mineralocorticoid excess (SAME), 11ßHSD is deficient, and cortisol is thus able to act as a mineralocorticoid, causing hypokalemic hypertension with a low renin and aldosterone. Excessive liquorice consumption can result in the same appearance. The active component of liquorice blocks 11ßHSD.

A similar pattern occurs in Liddle's syndrome in which the sodium channel in the distal tubule is persistently open and no longer governed by aldosterone. This mutant channel is sensitive to amiloride, which will ameliorate the hypertension.

Glucocorticoid sensitive hyperaldosteronism has a similar biochemical profile, and arises from a mutation that results in an abnormal enzyme with aldosterone synthase activity that is sensitive to adrenocorticotrophic hormone (ACTH). The result is an excess of mineralocorticoid activity and hypokalemic hypertension.

Other enzymatic mutations result in abnormal mineralocorticoid metabolism, such as 11ß hydroxylase deficiency and 17α hydroxylase deficiency. All these syndromes are rare, but provide an insight into how hypertension might be mediated in the wider population.

Oral contraceptives

Few medications have attracted more adverse publicity or more intense scrutiny than the combined oral contraceptive (OC) pill. The pill does increase the risk of cardiovascular disease, but this has to be seen in the context of a very low background risk of cardiovascular disease in young women. The risk is clearly related to increasing age of the patient, obesity, hypertension, and whether the patient smokes.

Most women taking the combined oral contraceptive have a small rise in blood pressure, amounting to hypertension in approximately 5%.[2] The incidence of hypertension rises with the duration of use. Blood pressure returns to normal in 50-60% of women when stopping the pill, but in the remainder, blood pressure remains elevated. It is unclear whether these women have contraceptive induced hypertension, or essential hypertension revealed by oral contraceptive use.

The OC should be prescribed with caution to women over the age of 35 who smoke. In the remainder, blood pressure should be measured six monthly. If hypertension is detected, the OC should be stopped and an alternative contraceptive used. Blood pressure should continue to be monitored to ensure that it returns to normal, or to allow early treatment if blood pressure remains elevated.

Pregnancy-induced hypertension is covered in Chapter 11.

Congenital renal disease

Many congenital renal syndromes are associated with hypertension, but raised blood pressure is rarely the presenting problem. An exception is polycystic renal disease. Adult polycystic disease is a dominantly inherited condition, present in approximately 1:1000 of the general population. The commonest presentation is with loin pain. Hematuria and hypertension also occur. The kidneys are always palpable except in the very obese, and the diagnosis is confirmed by renal ultrasound. There is no specific treatment for polycystic disease. Renal replacement therapy may become necessary as renal function deteriorates.

Management of hypertension in the young

Having made the diagnosis of hypertension in the young, a thorough examination is mandatory and should include an abdominal examination for the kidneys and renal bruits and a check for radio-femoral delay. The urine should be dipsticked.

Routine investigations should include an electrocardiogram and urea and electrolytes. Further investigations will be governed by the clinical situation; routine imaging of the renal tract is not indicated.

Before starting treatment, it is important to remember what the purpose of treatment is; that is, to prevent the complications of hypertension. This is particularly important in the young. Most of these patients will have essential hypertension, and the diagnosis of hypertension sentences them to a lifetime of treatment. For example, a young woman with a blood pressure of 150/95, while she might have a higher risk of cerebrovascular disease than her contemporaries, still has a very low *absolute* risk of complications, and it may not be in her interests to treat her blood pressure unless there is evidence of end-organ damage. Compliance can also be a particular problem in adolescence, and particularly where side-effects occur, such as impotence on ß-blockers.

References

1. The 1993 report of the Joint National Committee on detection evaluation and treatment of high blood pressure. *Arch Intern Med* 1993;153:154

2. Royal College of General Practitioners' oral contraception study. Further analyses of mortality in oral contraceptive users. *Lancet* 1981;1:541

Structural	Coarctation of the aorta
	Renal artery stenosis
Drugs	Oral contraceptives
	Steroids
	Liquorice
Renal disease	Polycystic kidneys
	Pyelonephritis
Hormonal	Cushing's syndrome
	Hyperparathyroidism
	Pheochromocytoma
Genetic	SAME *
	Alport's syndrome
	Glucocorticoid suppressible hyperaldoseronism
Miscellaneous	Neuroblastoma
	Lead poisoning

Table 1. *Some causes of hypertension in the young. *SAME is the syndrome of apparent mineralocorticoid excess.*

CHAPTER 10

HYPERTENSION, RENAL AND AUTOIMMUNE DISEASE *Neal Padmanabhan and Adrian Brady*

Introduction

Hypertension and the kidney are inextricably linked. Guyton argued that renal dysfunction, as either a primary or a secondary event, is necessary to produce a permanent rise in blood pressure. He called this the "overriding role of the kidney on blood pressure."[1] As well as being the cause of hypertension, renal failure may also be its consequence.

The incidence of End Stage Renal Failure (ESRF) is increasing in both Europe and the USA. Data from the United States Renal Data System (US RDS) indicated that 30% of all new cases of ESRF in 1992 had hypertension as a primary cause.[2] While the relevance of this data to other populations is questionable, there is no doubt that hypertension is an important risk factor for progressive renal failure. In this review we shall briefly discuss the relationship between the kidney and both essential and secondary hypertension, introduce the concept of renal failure as a predictor of cardiovascular risk and consider treatment options in hypertensive patients with renal failure.

1. The Kidney and Essential Hypertension: Culprit and Victim

Several lines of evidence suggest that the kidneys contribute to the development of essential hypertension. The most persuasive is from experiments demonstrating that transplantation of kidneys from genetically hypertensive rats to normotensive strains induces hypertension in the recipient.[3] Moreover, in humans recipients of kidneys from donors with a hypertensive background required significantly more anti-hypertensive medication than patients receiving "normotensive" kidneys.[4] Such observations suggest that a large part of the genetic predisposition to hypertension is enacted through the kidney.

As well as being a "culprit" in the etiology of hypertension, the kidney is also a "victim". Estimates of the incidence of chronic renal failure (CRF) in patients with essential hypertension vary. Untreated hypertension certainly results in CRF in a proportion of patients. Thus, in one series of 500 patients with hypertension, CRF was present in 18% and proteinuria in 42% at the time of death.[5] Since the advent of effective anti-hypertensive therapies, the risk of CRF associated with an elevated blood pressure has fallen. However, since hypertension is common, even a small risk may still represent a considerable burden of disease.

A recent projection suggested that 7.7% of hypertensives in the USA will develop CRF.[6] Prospective data obtained in 332,554 men screened for inclusion in the Multiple Risk Factor Intervention Trial (MRFIT) showed a graded relationship between the risk of ESRF and both baseline systolic and diastolic blood pressure.[7] Thus the risk of ESRF was increased 22-fold in patients with systolic pressures of $\geq$ 220 mmHg or diastolic pressures of $\geq$ 120 mmHg, compared to those with pressure of < 120/80 mmHg respectively. Most of the excess risk was attributable to systolic blood pressure.

The relationship between blood pressure and renal risk is modified by a number of factors. These include race, diabetes and proteinuria. African-Americans and Pacific Islanders account for a disproportionate number of people reaching ESRF in the USA. Moreover the pattern of renal disease in these populations is different from that seen in Caucasians. Data from the US RDS suggest that between 1990 and 1993, hypertension was the underlying cause of renal disease in 40% of African-American patients presenting for treatment with ESRF, compared with 27% in white patients.[1] In the UK the same may be true for patients of South Asian origin.

Another factor that modifies the relationship between blood pressure and renal failure is diabetes. In diabetes the relationship between renal risk, hypertension and proteinuria is complex. In type I diabetes, hypertension accompanies nephropathy and is associated with proteinuria (urine albumin excretion >300mg/24 hrs). Ultimately about 30% of patients with type 1 diabetes will develop hypertension.[8] There is also a transition phase with the presence of microalbuminuria (urine albumin excretion 30-300mg/24 hrs), during which elevation of blood pressure is unusual. In Type 2 diabetes there is frequently simultaneous essential hypertension and diabetes. Since the prevalence of obesity and hypertension increase with age, an association between these problems and diabetes is not surprising. However, the association holds after adjustment for age and weight and the risk of diabetic complications, including cardiovascular disease is strongly associated with blood pressure.[9]

2. Kidney disease and hypertension: pathophysiology
The relationship between renal failure and hypertension is complex. There are two related issues: how does CRF cause hypertension and how does hypertension, once established, contribute to the progression of CRF?

Renal causative mechanisms

The principal pathophysiological factors implicated in the generation of hypertension in patients with renal disease are as follows:

- Sodium and volume overload

- Neuroendocrine activation – principally the renin-angiotensin-aldosterone system (RAAS). Other vasoactive agents implicated include endothelin (ET), natriuretic peptides and possibly adrenomedullin.

- Sympathetic nervous system activation.

These factors are not mutually exclusive, but are intimately inter-related. There is considerable evidence that volume overload occurs very early in the course of renal disease, before hypertension is detected. One study investigated the relationship between circulating blood volume and central and peripheral hemodynamics in 97 patients with early parenchymal renal disease.[10] These patients had well-maintained renal function (GFR ~ 91 – 124 ml/min) and were either normotensive or had mild-to-moderate hypertension. A group of 13/32 normotensive patients were found to be "hyperkinetic," with an increased circulating blood volume, increased cardiac output

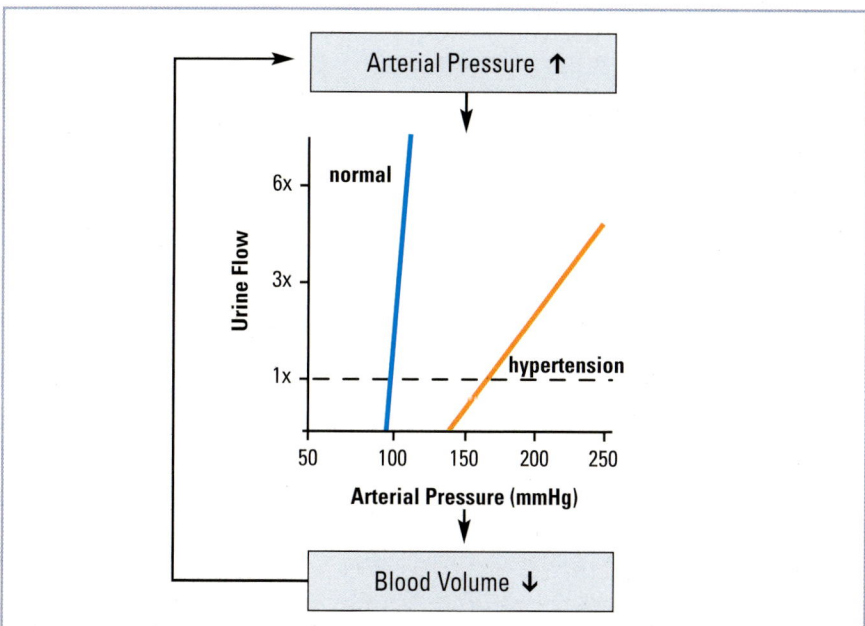

Figure 1. The pressure natriuretic response and regulation of blood pressure.

and reduced peripheral vascular resistance. After 2-8 years of follow-up 11 of these 12 patients had become hypertensive. The authors' conclusion was that the earliest abnormality was an increased circulating volume and cardiac output. However, a compensatory reduction in peripheral resistance maintained normotension. When this adaptation ceased blood pressure rose and blood volume normalized, possibly by induction of a pressure natriuresis.

The concept of pressure natriuresis is fundamental to an understanding of the renal regulation of extracellular fluid (ECF) volume, sodium balance and blood pressure. The renal response to arterial hypertension is to increase sodium and water excretion, in order to return blood pressure to normal.[1] Hypertension results when the pressure-natriuretic response is shifted to maintain sodium balance at higher levels of blood pressure – see Figure 1.

As blood pressure increases, the kidney compensates by increasing sodium and water excretion, so reducing extracellular volume and hence blood pressure. Steady state at a given blood pressure is achieved when sodium intake and excretion are equal. In hypertension sodium intake is matched by excretion, but at a higher level of blood pressure. From Cowley et al [11]

Activation of the RAAS is also regarded as an important factor influencing the renal regulation of blood pressure. Early studies in patients with ESRF suggested that renin secretion was excessive in relation to the degree of sodium retention and ECF volume overload.[10] The same may also be true of plasma renin activity (PRA) in early renal failure. Here, a normal PRA in the context of ECF volume increase could be interpreted as an inappropriate failure of suppression of the RAAS.[12] In-vitro evidence also supports the notion that the RAAS is involved in both the short and long term regulation of blood pressure.

Angiotensin II (Ang II) is a systemic and renal vasoconstrictor and promotes tubular sodium reabsorption directly and through aldosterone. In addition it upregulates local vasoactive agents such as ET and interacts with growth factors such as TGFß.[13-15]

In addition to neuroendocrine activation, there is also evidence for direct neurogenic regulation of blood pressure in patients with CRF. Sympathetic over-activity has been demonstrated in patients with CRF and may therefore represent a response to renal injury.[16]

Hypertension and chronic renal failure

Figure 2 illustrates in schematic form the relationship between hypertension and progression of CRF. It is thought that the crucial abnormality is the exposure of the glomerulus to systemic blood pressure. This may be due either to inappropriate afferent arteriolar vasodilation, or efferent vasoconstriction. Glomerular hypertension in turn leads to endothelial damage and activation of pro-fibrotic paracrine mediators. Glomerulosclerosis results and the reduction in nephron numbers induces compensatory hyperfiltration and perpetuates the process. Consistent with this hypothesis, Schmeider et al showed that patients with essential hypertension and high glomerular filtration rates (GFR) had the most rapid loss of renal function. [17]

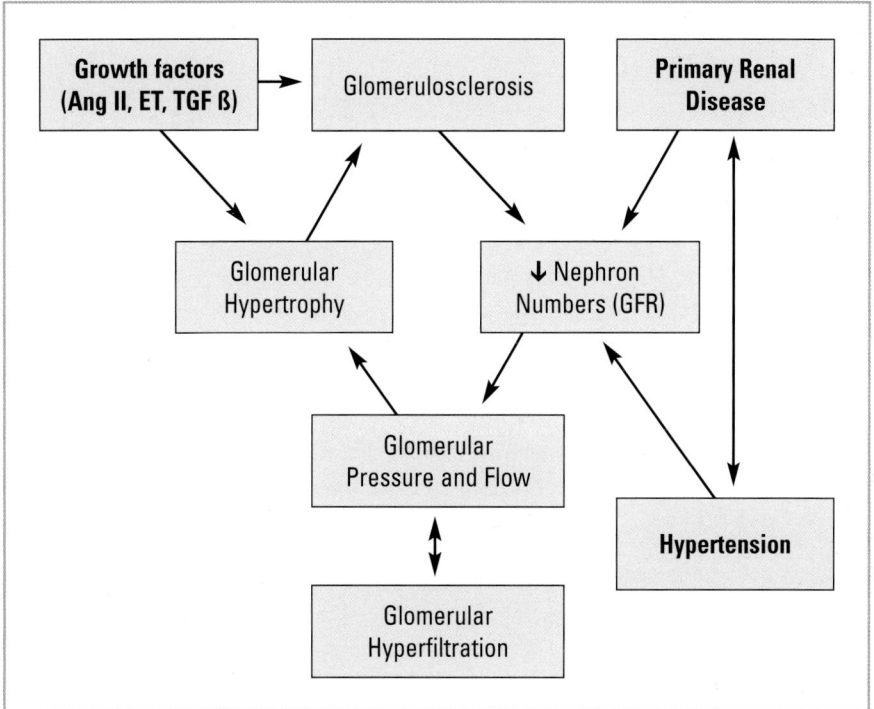

Figure 2. The circle of hypertension and glomerulosclerosis

3. The Kidney and Secondary Hypertension
CRF is almost always accompanied by hypertension. Hence the renal differential diagnosis of secondary hypertension is effectively that of chronic renal failure itself.

● **Vascular causes:**
  Vascular disease affecting the kidney may be either acute or chronic. Acute causes include vasculitis, malignant hypertension and scleroderma. The most important chronic cause is atherosclerotic renovascular disease. This is an important and increasing cause of CRF in Western populations. Recent estimates suggest that 5-25% of patients presenting with ESRF have renovascular disease.[18]

Patients with peripheral vascular disease are at particularly high risk. One study of 100 consecutive patients presenting with peripheral vascular disease identified 24 patients with bilateral renal artery stenosis and seven patients with a renal artery occlusion.[19] Atherosclerotic renovascular disease should be suspected in patients with severe or refractory hypertension, CRF and evidence of vascular disease elsewhere. Some patients may present with pulmonary oedema with normal left ventricular function – "flash pulmonary edema" – or an increase in creatinine after administration of an ACE-inhibitor. Urinalysis is usually normal, though proteinuria does occur if secondary focal glomerulosclerosis has developed. Ultrasound may reveal asymmetric renal size. Diagnosis increasingly relies on magnetic resonance angiography.

Glomerular Disease

Glomerular disease may be due to idiopathic primary renal disease or occur as part of a systemic disorder. There are two main patterns of presentation, with considerable overlap. The nephritic syndrome comprises renal impairment, hypertension and edema. Urinalysis reveals an active sediment with dysmorphic red cells, white cells and granular and cellular casts. Such patients will usually have a diffuse glomerulonephritis, such as might occur with lupus nephritis, post-infectious glomerulonephritis (GN) or ANCA-associated GN.

Rapidly Progressive Glomerulonephritis (RPGN)

Although rare, it is crucially important to recognize patients who might have rapidly progressive GN (RPGN). RPGN may present with the nephritic syndrome, but frequently has a prodromal phase associated with symptoms such as malaise, arthropathy, epistaxis, nasal stuffiness and hemoptysis, followed by rapidly declining renal function. Renal failure can develop very quickly in these patients, and once oligo-anuria has ensued, is not always reversible. Such patients may benefit from early aggressive immunosuppressive therapy with high-dose corticosteroids, cyclophosphamide and (in some regimes) plasmapheresis. Diagnosis requires a renal biopsy which will reveal a necrotizing glomerulonephritis, with crescent formation.

The pattern of immunofluorescence (IF) may also be informative. For example the presence of linear IgG deposition, as occurs in Goodpasture's disease (associated with anti-GGM antibodies) or the absence of immuno-staining ("pauci-immune") which may indicate Wegener's Granulomatosis or Microscopic Polyangiitis (associated with anti PR3 or MPO antibodies, respectively). Many patients, however, have focal disease (less than 50% of glomeruli involved). Such patients have a more benign presentation. The most common primary glomerular disorder in the UK is IgA Nephropathy, which usually causes a focal GN. This disorder is characterized by persistent microscopic hematuria, frequently with proteinuria, and approximately 1/3 of patients develop ESRF. Bouts of macroscopic haematuria may follow upper respiratory tract infections.

The nephrotic syndrome comprises heavy proteinuria (>3g/24 hours), peripheral edema, hypoalbuminuria and hyperlipidemia. The differential diagnosis of the nephrotic syndrome varies considerably with the age of the patient. Children and young adults will most commonly have minimal change disease and will be normotensive, with preserved renal function.

Older patients are more likely to have focal segmental glomerulosclerosis (FSGS) or membranous GN. Diabetic nephropathy is an important secondary cause of the nephrotic syndrome, as is primary amyloidosis (which may be related to the presence of multiple myeloma, but may also occur independently). In one study of 233 patients who presented with nephrotic syndrome 33% of patients had membranous GN, 33% had FSGS, 15% had minimal change disease and 4% had amyloidosis (but 10% in those aged > 44 years).[20]

- **Tubulo-Interstitial Disease**
  By far the most common tubular disorder causing renal failure is acute tubular necrosis (ATN), which may occur after any ischemic insult to the kidney. Other tubular disorders that may present acutely include acute interstitial nephritis (most frequently related to antibiotics or non-steroidal anti-inflammatories) and cast nephropathy, due to myeloma. Chronic tubulo-interstitial diseases include chronic pyelonephritis, analgesic nephropathy and polycystic kidney disease.

- **Obstructive uropathy**
  This may occur due to obstruction of the urinary tract anywhere below the renal pelvis. Clinically detectable (by measurement of serum creatinine) renal impairment usually requires bilateral upper tract obstruction to be present. In older patients malignancy is a frequent cause. It is important to realize that obstruction may be present even where urine output is preserved and should always be excluded as a cause of unexplained renal failure.

Investigation of Renal Disease
Assessment of renal structure and function is mandatory in patients with suspected secondary hypertension. A detailed drug and family history should be taken. Investigations should include serum urea and creatinine, urine microscopy for red cells and casts and dipstick tests for blood and protein. Proteinuria should be quantified by a 24-hour collection, with estimation of creatinine clearance. Renal ultrasound may indicate if there has been chronic renal damage, will identify polycystic kidney disease and exclude obstruction.

Renal scintigraphy can be both static (using ^{99m}Tc labeled DMSA to investigate split renal function and show renal scarring, as might be present in chronic pyelonephritis); and dynamic (using ^{99m}Tc labeled DTPA, or MAG-3, to investigate renal perfusion and excretion). Renal angiography is the gold-standard for the diagnosis of renal artery stenosis, although MR angiography is becoming more readily available. Screening tests for glomerular and associated systemic disease might include anti-streptolysin O (ASO) titres, autoantibodies (e.g. ANF, dsDNA, ANCA, GBM), complement studies, hepatitis titres and both serum and urine electrophoresis.

4. Hypertension, Renal Disease and Cardiovascular Risk

Renal impairment is associated with a huge increase in the risk of cardiovascular disease, which accounts for up to 50% of all deaths in patients with CRF or ESRF. The relative increase in risk is largest in young patients. In the USA cardiac mortality in dialysis patients < 45 years is 100 times greater than in the general population – see figure 3.[21] The major structural cardiovascular abnormality found in patients with ESRF is left ventricular hypertrophy (LVH), which is found in 75% of patients commencing dialysis.[22] Clinical evidence of cardiac failure is found in 33% of new dialysis patients, angina in 25% and a history of myocardial infarction in 10%.[23]

Not only are patients with renal failure more likely to experience cardiovascular disease, but their prognosis from it is worse than other populations. Thus, the one year mortality after acute myocardial infarction in dialysis patients in the USA was found to be 59% (and even greater in diabetic patients with ESRF).[24]

One issue that is currently the subject of much debate is whether uremia itself is a cardiac risk factor. The demonstration of a high incidence of cardiovascular disease in patients with renal failure does not prove that CRF *causes* cardiovascular disease. The association might also arise because cardiovascular disease causes renal

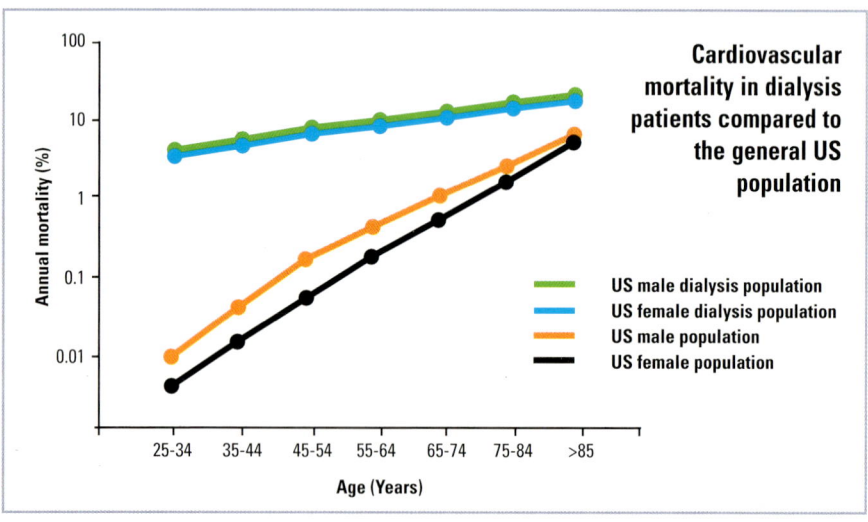

Figure 3. Cardiac mortality in dialysis patients.

dysfunction, or because other risk factors, such as hyperlipidemia, hypertension or diabetes (or other, unidentified, risk factors) predispose patients to *both* renal failure *and* cardiovascular disease. A detailed discussion of the possible contributions of various risk factors to the increased incidence of cardiovascular disease seen in renal failure is beyond the scope of this article, but is well reviewed by Baigent at al.[25]

Microalbuminuria (MAL: urine albumin excretion 30-300mg/24 hrs) is present in 20-30% of non-diabetic hypertensives.[26] It is a marker for both high cardiovascular risk and progressive renal failure, but has yet to be established as an independent risk factor per se in these subjects.[27]

5. Treatment of Hypertension in Patients with Renal Disease

The two main issues in the treatment of hypertension in patients with renal impairment are (1) the degree of blood pressure reduction that is desirable and (2) the choice of anti-hypertensive agent to be used. Most guidelines currently suggest that blood pressure should be reduced to < 140/85 mmHg. However the Modification of Diet in Renal Disease (MDRD) study suggested that the blood pressure target in patients with proteinuria of > 1 g/24 hrs should be 125/75 mmHg.[28] This is based on epidemiological studies rather than randomized controlled trials, which suggest that there is no blood pressure threshold for the risk of progression of renal disease. Thus, a recent consensus statement (JNC VI) suggested a target of 130/85 in diabetes, or 125/75 mmHg in the presence of proteinuria of ≥ 1g/24 hrs.[29]

The benefits of aggressive blood pressure reduction in diabetics were emphasized by the results of the Hypertension Optimal Therapy (HOT) Trial.[30] The lowest risk of major cardiovascular events was at a DBP of 82.6 mmHg. In the subgroup with diabetes there was a significant reduction in cardiovascular mortality in the < 80 mmHg subgroup.

The choice of antihypertensive agent is still much debated. While the degree of blood pressure reduction is clearly important, it is often asserted that ACEIs - and angiotensin receptor antagonists (ARBs) - have additional blood pressure-independent actions. These claims are often based on surrogate end-points rather than actual disease states or events. However, a number of studies have demonstrated that ACEIs slow the progression of chronic renal disease, and are particularly effective in the presence of proteinuria.

ACEIs reduce intra-glomerular pressure, reduce filtration fraction and increase GFR. In addition ACEIs also reduce mesangial cell proliferation and matrix production. The Collaborative Study Group showed in patients with Type I Diabetes and proteinuria of ≥ 0.5g/24 hrs, that treatment with captopril was associated with a reduction in the risk of a doubling of serum creatinine of 48% compared with conventional therapy.[31] In non-diabetic renal disease benazepril had a similar effect, reducing the risk of a doubling of creatinine, or ESRF, by 53%.[32]

Treatment with ACEI reduces proteinuria to a greater extent than other agents. The effect of ACEIs on the progression of renal failure in proteinuric patients was studied by the GISEN group.[33] In this study ramipril or placebo was given in addition to conventional therapy in patients with proteinuria of either 1-3 g/24 hrs (Stratum 1), or ≥ 3g/24 hrs (Stratum 2). Treatment with ramipril was highly effective in Stratum 2 and the trial was prematurely terminated for these patients because of this.

ARBs are a new class of drugs with a good side effect profile. There are also a number of theoretical reasons why ARBs may be at least equivalent to or possibly superior than ACE-inhibitors – for example angiotensin II generation by non-ACE pathways.[34] They appear to have similar actions to ACEIs on renal hemodynamics and proteinuria. A number of recent trials have examined the effects of ARBs in patients with diabetic nephropathy.

The RENAAL study investigated the use of losartan in 1513 patients with type 2 diabetes.[35] Patients with urinary albumin excretion of > 300 mg/l or total protein excretion of ≥ 0.5g/24 hours were randomized to receive losartan or placebo in addition to standard anti-hypertensive therapy (not including ACE-inhibitors) and followed for a mean of 3.4 years. Losartan reduced the risk of the primary composite end-point of doubling of serum creatinine, ESRF or death by 16%. There was a marked renoprotective effect, with a highly significant reduction in the risk of ESRF of 28%.

Another study compared the effects of the ARB, irbesartan with amlodipine or placebo in patients with type II diabetes and nephropathy.[36] Here, treatment with an ARB was associated with a reduction in the risk of a doubling of serum creatinine of 33% and ESRF of 23%. Compared to irbesartan, and for an equivalent blood pressure control, amlodipine had no renoprotective effect.

No trials have directly compared ARBs with ACEIs in terms of their renoprotective effects, but there has been interest in the possibility of combining the two classes of drugs. It has been hypothesized that greater inhibition of the RAAS will bring about greater benefits. This strategy is under investigation in patients with heart failure, where the benefits of dual blockade have been found to be equivocal.

In renal disease there have been a few small studies. Mogensen et al studied patients with hypertension, type 2 diabetes and MAL who were randomized to receive candesartan, lisinopril or combination.[37] A significant reduction of both blood pressure and albuminuria was observed in patients treated with the combination. A further small study in patients with IgA nephropathy demonstrated a significant additive (and blood pressure-independent) reduction in proteinuria when losartan and enalapril were used together.[38] Long-term outcome studies of combination therapy in renal disease are, however, awaited.

The use of calcium channel blockers (CCBs) in renal disease is controversial. There is no doubt that CCBs are effective anti-hypertensive agents – as demonstrated for example by the HOT, Syst-Eur and Insight studies. However, CCBs preferentially vasodilate the afferent arteriole, allowing greater transmission of systemic blood pressure to the glomerulus. Thus, it is possible that the benefit of systemic blood pressure reduction is offset by a smaller reduction in glomerular hypertension and thus less renoprotection.

A recent meta-analysis suggested that ACEIs and non-dihydropyridine CCBs induced a greater reduction in proteinuria than nifedipine, and that, for ACEIs at least, this was associated with greater preservation of GFR.[39] Since the pharmacological effects of CCBs – to vasodilate afferent arterioles – and ACEIs – to vasodilate efferent arterioles are complementary, it is possible that their combination should significantly reduce intra-glomerular pressure and have a synergistic renoprotective effect. A recent prospective study in patients with type 2 diabetes tested this hypothesis and showed that, while both verapamil and lisinopril reduced proteinuria, there was indeed evidence of synergy when they were used in combination.[40]

Diuretics are important in the treatment of chronic renal failure, especially if volume overload develops. As CRF progresses thiazide diuretics become ineffective and loop diuretics are required to achieve a significant natriuresis and reduction in extracellular volume. There is, however, no evidence that diuretic therapy slows the progression of renal disease.

ß-blockers are not generally considered to be first-line agents in the treatment of hypertension in patients with renal impairment but are frequently indicated by the presence of ischemic heart disease. However, the UKPDS study of patients with type 2 diabetes suggested similar efficacy of captopril and atenolol in the prevention of microvascular or macrovascular endpoints when blood pressure was tightly controlled.[41] There is no such equivalence in non-diabetic renal disease.

In conclusion, theoretical considerations and limited evidence suggest that ACEIs are the treatment of choice in hypertensive patients with CRF, especially if proteinuria is evident. If ACEIs are not tolerated, ARBs may be the best alternative; and combination therapy is an attractive future prospect. In clinical practice, adequate control is rarely achieved with ACEI monotherapy and multiple drugs are required. In this situation the addition of a CCB to an ACEI is logical, as is diuretic therapy, which potentiates the effect of the ACEI by inducing sodium depletion. If further therapy is required either a ß or an α-blocker may be added. Many patients will require multiple drug therapy.

Renal diagnosis	Clinical Presentation	Investigations
Primary Glomerular Disease		
● IgA Nephropathy	Hematuria, urinary casts, proteinuria	Immunoglobulins
● Mesangiocapillary glomerulonephritis	Hematuria, proteinuria, partial lipodystrophy	Exclude other causes (SLE, Hepatitis C, Cryoglobulinemia); Complement, C3 nephritic factor
● Membranous glomerulonephritis	Nephrotic syndrome	Gold therapy, malignancy, infections e.g. malaria
● Diffuse or Rapidly progressive glomerulonephritis	Nephritic syndrome, post infectious GN,	ASO titres, Autoantibodies (dsDNA, ANF, cANCA, pANCA, GBM), Complement,
● Focal segmental glomerulosclerosis	Nephrotic syndrome	
Glomerulonephritis secondary to Systemic Disease		
● SLE	Nephritic or nephrotic + extra-renal features	Complement, Autoantibodies – especially dsDNA
● Systemic Necrotizing Vasculitides: Wegener's granulomatosis, Microscopic polyangiitis, Churg-Strauss syndrome	Features of systemic disease e.g. malaise, polyarthropathy, nasal stuffiness, epistaxis, pulmonary hemorrhage, nephritic syndrome	ANCA, GBM, Complement
● Anti-GBM Disease	Pulmonary-renal syndrome	GBM antibody
Renal Artery Stenosis	widespread vascular disease, diabetes, pulmonary edema	MRA, CT angiography, arteriography
Congenital Renal disease	Family history	Ultrasound Scan
● Polycystic Kidney Disease	ultrasound appearances, sub-arachnoid hemorrhage	
● Alport's Syndrome	deafness, ocular manifestations, male sex	Biopsy
Chronic Pyelonephritis/Reflux Nephropathy	history of recurrent UTIs and Vesico-Ureteric Reflux	Ultrasound scan, DMSA

This is not an exhaustive list, but encompasses most of the common renal causes of hypertension.

Table 1. Renal causes of secondary hypertension.

Summary

● Chronic renal failure is both a cause and consequence of hypertension

● Renal disease is an important cause of secondary hypertension. Hypertensive patients should be screened for renal impairment and referred to a Renal Unit for investigation if present.

● Chronic renal failure is a state of high cardiovascular risk.

● Aggressive anti-hypertensive treatment may retard the progression of chronic renal failure.

● ACEIs are used as first line agents in patients with CRF and hypertension. They should be commenced as early as possible and titrated up to the highest tolerated dose, taking care to monitor electrolytes and creatinine.

● ARBs are used as first line agents in patients with hypertension, diabetes and proteinuria

● Monotherapy is rarely effective when there is significant renal impairment.

References

1. Guyton AC, Hall JE, Coleman TJ, Manning RDJ. The dominant role of the kidneys in the long-term regulation of arterial pressure in normal hypertensive states. In Hypertension: Pathophysiology, Diagnosis and Management. Edited by Laragh GH and Brenner BM. Raven Press: New York; 1990, 1029-1052.

2. US Renal Data System. USRDS 1996 Annual Data Report. Bethesda MD. National Institutes of Health, National Institute of Diabetes and Digestive and Kidney Diseases 1996.

3. Rettig R, Strauss H, Folberth C, Ganten D, Waldherr R, Unger T. Hypertension transmitted by kidneys from stroke-prone spontaneously hypertensive rats. Am J Physiol 1989; 257: F197-F203 Guidi E, Menghetti D, Milani S, Montagnino G, Palazzi P, Bianchi G. Hypertension may be transplanted with the kidney in humans. A long-term historical prospective follow-up of recipients grafted with kidneys coming from donors with or without hypertension in their families. J Am Soc Nephrol 1996; 7: 1131-1138.

5. Perera GA. Hypertensive vascular disease: description and natural history. J Chronic Dis 1955; 1: 33-42.

6. Perneger TV, Klag MJ, Felman HI, Whelton PK. Projections of hypertension-related renal disease in middle aged residents of the United States. JAMA 1993; 269: 1272-1277.

7. Klag MJ, Whelton PK, Randall BL, Neaton JD, Brancati FL, Ford CE, Shulman NB, Stamler J. A prospective study of blood pressure and incidence of end-stage renal disease in 332,544 men. N Engl J Med 1996;334, 13-18.

8. Mathiesen ER, Ronn B, Jensen T, Stroem B, Deckert T. Relationship between blood pressure and urinary albumin excretion in development of microalbuminuria. Diabetes 1990; 39: 245-249.

9. Adler AI, Stratton IM, Neil HA, Yudkin JS, Matthews DR, Cull CA, Wright AD, Turner RC, Holman RR. Association of systolic blood pressure with macrovascular and microvascular complications of type 2 diabetes (UKPDS 36): prospective observational study. BMJ 2000; 321: 412-419.

10. Brod J, Bahlman J, Cachovan M, Pretschner P. Development of hypertension in renal disease. Clin Sci 1983; 64: 141-152.

11. Cowley AW, Mattison DL, Lu S, Roman RJ. The renal medulla and hypertension. Hypertension 1995; 25: 663-673.

12. Schalekamp MADG, Schalekamp-Kuyken MPA, deFloor-Fruytier M, Menget T, Vaandrager-Kranenburg DJ, Birkenhager WH. Interrelationships between blood pressure, renin, renin substrate and blood volume in terminal renal failure. Clin Soc Mol Med 1973; 45: 417-428

13. Wolf G, Mueller E, Stahl RAK, Ziyadeh FN. Angiotensin II-induced hypertrophy of cultured murine proximal tubular cells is mediated by endogenous transforming growth factor-b. J Clin Invest 1993; 92: 1366-1372.

14. Bakris GL, Re RN. Endothelin modulates angiotensin II-induced mitogenesis of human mesangial cells. Am J Physiol 1993; 264: F937-942.

15. Wolf G, Zahner G, Schroeder R, Stahl RAK. Transforming growth factor beta mediates the angiotensin II-induced stimulation of collagen type IV synthesis in cultured murine proximal tubular cells. Nephrol Dial Transplant 1996; 11: 263-269

16. Converse RL, Jacobsen TN, Toto RD, Jost CMT, Cosentino F, Fouad-Tarazi F, Victor RG. Sympathetic overactivity in patients with CRF. New Eng J Med 1992; 327: 1912-1918.

17. Schmieder RE, Veelken R, Gatzka CD, Ruddel H, Schachinger H. J Hypertens 1995; 13: 357-365.

18. Rimmer JM, Gennari FJ. Atherosclerotic renovascular disease and progressive renal failure. Ann Intern Med 1993; 118: 712-719.

19. Choudri AH, Cleland JG, Rowlands PL. Unsuspected renal artery stenosis in peripheral vascular disease. BMJ 1990; 301: 1197.

20. Haas M, Meehan SM, Karrison TG, Spargo BH. Changing etiologies of unexplained adult nephrotic syndrome. A comparison of renal biopsy findings from 1976-1979 and 1995-1997. Am J Kid Dis 1997; 30 : 621-631.

21. Foley RN, Parfrey PS, Sarnak MJ. Clinical epidemiology of cardiovascular disease in chronic renal disease. Am J Kid Dis 1998; 32 (suppl 3): S112-119.

22. London GM, Marchais SJ, Guerin AP, Metivier F, Pannier B. Cardiac hypertrophy and arterial alterations in end-stage renal disease; haemodynamic factors. Kidney Int 1993; 43: S42-49.

23. US Renal Data System. 1999 Annual Data Report. Bethesda: National Institutes of Health, National Institute of Diabetes and Digestive and Kidney Diseases, April 1999.

24. Herzog CA, Jennie Z, Collins AJ. Poor long-term survival after acute myocardial infarction among patients on long -term dialysis. N Engl J Med 1998; 339, 799-805.
Baigent C, Burbury K, Wheeler D. Premature cardiovascular disease in chronic renal failure. Lancet 2000;356: 147-152.

26. Agrawal B, Berger A, Wolf K, Luft FC. Microalbuminuria screening by reagent strip predicts cardiovascular risk in hypertension. J Hypertens 1996; 14:: 223-228.

27. Bianchi S, Bigazzi R, Campese VM. Microalbuminuria in essential hypertension: significance, pathophysiology and therapeutic implications. Am J Kid Dis 1999; 34: 973-995.

28. Peterson JC, Adler S, Burkart JM, Greene T, Hebert LA, Hunsicker LG et al, for the Modification of Diet in Renal Disease (MDRD) Study Group. Blood pressure control, proteinuria and the progression of renal disease. The Modification of Diet in Renal Disease Study. Ann Intern Med 1995; 123: 754-762.

29. Joint National Committee on Prevention, Detection, Evaluation and Treatment of High Blood Pressure: The Sixth Report of the Joint National Committee on Prevention, Detection, Evaluation and Treatment of High Blood Pressure (JNC VI). Arch Int Med 1997; 157: 2413-2446.

30. Hansson L, Zanchetti A, Carruthers SG, Dahlof B, Elmfeldt D, Julius S, Menard J, Rahn KH, Wedel H, Westerling S. Effects of intensive blood pressure lowering and low-dose aspirin in patients with hypertension. Principal results of the Hypertension Optimal Treatment (HOT) randomised trial. Lancet 1998; 351: 1755-1762.

31. Lewis EJ, Hunsicker LG, Bain DP, Rohde RD. The effect of angiotensin-converting enzyme inhibition on diabetic nephropathy. New Eng J Med 1993; 329: 1456-1462.

32. Maschio G, Alberti D, Janin G, Locatelli F, Mann JFE, Motolese M, et al, on behalf of the ACE inhibition in progressive renal disease stud group. Effect of the angiotensin-converting-enzyme -inhibitor benazepril on the progression of chronic renal insufficiency. New Eng J Med 1996; 334: 939-945.

33. The Gisen group (Gruppo Italiano di Studi epidemilogici in Nefrologia). Randomised placebo-controlled trial of the effect of ramipril on decline in glomerular filtration rate and risk of terminal renal failure in protenuric, non-diabetic, nephropathy. Lancet 1997; 349: 1857-1863.

34. Padmanabhan N. Jardine AG. McGrath JC. Connell JMC. Angiotensin-converting enzyme independent contraction to angiotensin I in human resistance arteries. Circulation 1999; 99(22): 2914-2920.

35. Brenner BM, Cooper ME, de Zeeuw D, Keane WF, Mitch WE, Parving H-H, Remuzzi G, Snapinn SM, Zhang Z, Shahinfar S for the RENAAL Study Investigators. Effects of losartan on renal and cardiovascular outcomes in patients with type 2 diabetes and nephropathy. New Eng J Med 2001; 345: 861869.

36. Lewis EJ, Hunsicker LG, Clarke WR, Berl T, Pohl MA, Lewis JB, Ritz E, Atkins RC, Rohde R, Raz I for the Collaborative Study Group. Renoprotective effect of the angiotensin-receptor antagonist irbesartan in patients with nephropathy due to type 2 diabetes. New Eng J Med 2001; 345: 851-860.

37. Mogensen CE, Neldam S, Tikkanen I, Oren S, Viskoper R, watts RW, Cooper ME. Randomised trial of dual blockade of renin-angiotensin system in patients with hypertension, microalbuminuria and non-insulin dependent diabetes: the candesartan and lisinopril microalbuminuria (CALM) study. BMJ 2000; 321: 1440-1444.

38. Russo D, Minutolo R, Pisani A, Esposito R, Signoriello G, Andreucci M, Balleta MM. Co-administration of losartan and enalapril exerts additive antiproteinuric effect in IgA nephropathy. Am J Kid Dis 2001; 38: 18-25.

39. Weidmann P, Schneider M, Bohlen L. Therapeutic efficacy of different antihypertensive drugs in human diabetic nephropathy: an updated meta-analysis. Nephrol Dial Transplant 1995; 10 : S39-45

40. Lash JP, Bakris GL. Effects of ACE-inhibitors and calcium antagonists alone or combined on progression of diabetic nephropathy. Nephrol Dial Transplant 1995; 10: S56-62.

41. UK Prospective Diabetes Study Group. Efficacy of atenolol and captopril in reducing risk of macrovascular and microvascular complications in type 2 diabetes: UKPDS 39. BMJ 1998; 317: 713-720.

CHAPTER 11

HYPERTENSION IN PREGNANCY; ORAL CONTRACEPTIVES AND HORMONE REPLACEMENT THERAPY *Mary Joan MacLeod, Adrian Brady and Ian Greer*

Hypertension in pregnancy is a major cause of maternal death and perinatal morbidity and mortality. Many maternal deaths reflect substandard care both in the community and hospital setting. This includes a failure to recognize symptoms and signs, such as epigastric pain, headache and visual disturbance associated with severe disease, and a failure to adequately control hypertension. With regard to the former it is critical that any woman presenting with these symptoms in pregnancy have her blood pressure measured and urinalysis for protein performed.

Measuring blood pressure in pregnancy
Blood pressure normally decreases early in pregnancy, with mid-trimester diastolic pressure often 10 mmHg, or more, lower than pre-pregnancy levels, rising gradually towards non-pregnant values near term. As cardiac output increases by around 40% in the first trimester and is maintained through pregnancy, this must reflect a reduction in peripheral vascular resistance. Hypertension results from an increase in systemic vascular resistance in the face of an unchanged cardiac output.

Until recently, diastolic pressure in pregnancy was taken at the point when the sounds muffle (Korotkoff phase IV) rather than where they disappear (Korotkoff phase V). However, the assumption that the sounds never disappear in pregnant women appears to be unfounded[3] and phase V is again preferred as in non-pregnant individuals. Blood pressure should be measured with the woman sitting quietly, using an appropriately sized cuff, and the stethoscope bell lightly applied to the arm. Pressure should be measured to the nearest 2 mmHg.

Classifying hypertension in pregnancy

Hypertension in pregnancy can be classified as:

- preexisting or chronic

- gestational or pregnancy-induced hypertension (PIH) which can be mild/moderate (BP140-160/90-110mmHg) or severe (Systolic BP >160 or diastolic BP > 110mmHg)

- pre-eclampsia where PIH is associated with the development of new proteinuria.

In pregnancy, just as in the non-pregnant population, blood pressure is continuously distributed and the dividing line between normotension and hypertension is arbitrary and artificial. A diastolic blood pressure of 90 mmHg after 20 weeks of pregnancy is the threshold for diagnosis. There is merit in this as the perinatal mortality rate increases when diastolic blood pressure exceeds this level. In addition, it fits with statistical descriptions of blood pressure in the population. A diastolic pressure of 90 mmHg is 3 SD greater than the mean for mid-pregnancy, 2 SD above the mean for 34 weeks' gestation but only 1.5 SD above the mean at term, reflecting the physiological increase in blood pressure towards term.

In late pregnancy this can lead to over-diagnosis of hypertension and may precipitate unnecessary intervention. While in the late second trimester a 90mmHg threshold may lead to under-diagnosis. This threshold excludes women who have a substantial increase in blood pressure but where the diastolic pressure does not exceed 90 mmHg, and will include some women with chronic hypertension who have a minimal increase in pressure. Thus the increase in pressure from early pregnancy should also be considered. Repeated measures of blood pressure should be made to obtain an accurate diagnosis. Because of the diurnal variation and short term variability of blood pressure, multiple measures of blood pressure are required to obtain a true assessment of the situation.

Chronic (essential) hypertension

Chronic (essential) hypertension occurs in 1-5% of women of childbearing age, and can be diagnosed in pregnancy on the basis of known hypertension before pregnancy, or a pressure of greater than 140/90 mmHg before 20 weeks gestation. It may be present preconceptually, but diagnosed for the first time in pregnancy. These woman have a ten-fold increased risk (an incidence of around 20%) of developing superimposed PIH or preeclampsia. When pre-eclampsia does occur it is usually severe and early onset in nature and likely to recur in future pregnancies. Intrauterine fetal growth restriction (IUGR) is also more common.

Most of the excess morbidity associated with chronic hypertension relates to the development of superimposed pre-eclampsia. However, where the hypertension is secondary to a problem such as chronic renal disease a deterioration in the primary condition may occur in the absence of superimposed pre-eclampsia. Women with chronic hypertension at highest risk of developing superimposed pre-eclampsia are those with severe hypertension, a diastolic pressure of >100mmHg before 20 weeks gestation, and those with evidence of target organ damage such as left ventricular hypertrophy or renal compromise, where the risk of pre-eclampsia may be over 40%. Thus where chronic hypertension has been present for several years an assessment of target organ damage should be made.

With chronic hypertension it is often possible to discontinue antihypertensive therapy in the first half of pregnancy, as blood pressure shows the same physiological changes as in normal pregnancy, although it may require to be reintroduced in the third trimester as blood pressure rises from its physiological nadir in mid-pregnancy. Ambulatory blood pressure monitoring may be particularly useful in these women. Such treatment should be instituted if diastolic pressure is $\geq$ 100mmHg or 90mmHg if there is underlying renal disease or evidence of target organ damage. Ideally these women should be seen pre-pregnancy in order to review the level of risk, assess end organ damage and review antihypertensive therapy as some agents such as ACE inhibitors and AII receptor antagonists are best avoided in pregnancy.

Pregnancy induced hypertension (PIH) and Pre-eclampsia

PIH is the diagnosis applied to women who are normotensive in the first 20 weeks of pregnancy, but who develop hypertension in the second half of pregnancy. When Diastolic pressure is persistently between 90-110mmHg it is termed mild to moderate PIH and severe PIH if diastolic blood pressure is >110 mmHg. It should be noted that up to 20% of pregnant women will have at least one diastolic reading of $\geq$90mmHg. When proteinuria (>0.3g/24h) also occurs, regardless of whether the hypertension is mild/moderate or severe, it is termed pre-eclampsia. The disorder is not simply a problem of hypertension and renal dysfunction manifest as proteinuria. These are simply two clinical features of a complex multi-system condition with widespread endothelial dysfunction producing a variable systemic upset including disturbance of coagulation and hepatic function. The trigger for the condition lies within the placenta and may reflect abnormal implantation or an abnormally large placenta such as in twin pregnancy.

Prediction and prevention

Although we know many risk factors for pre-eclampsia such as obesity, family history, and high blood pressure in early pregnancy, we have, at least at present, no specific or sensitive enough test to determine pregnancies at high risk. The disturbance in placentation can be assessed by Doppler ultrasound arterial waveform analysis from the maternal uterine arteries in the second trimester. Such studies have shown an association between high-resistance waveform patterns and pre-eclampsia in high risk women, but this has limited accuracy in predicting pre-eclampsia in low risk women. Combinations of risk factors have also been used for prediction of pre-eclampsia. This might be most valuable when combined with biochemical risk markers. Low dose aspirin therapy is associated with a 15% reduction in the risk of pre-eclampsia associated with the use of antiplatelet agents, but further information is required to identify which women were most likely to benefit and when treatment should be started. In practical terms aspirin should be considered in the management of women with a history of severe or early onset preeclampsia or specific underlying medical conditions that place them at increase risk such as chronic hypertension, connective tissue or renal disease - it seems likely that these women should begin prophylactic treatment early in the second trimester or sooner if they have a problem such as antiphospholipid antibody syndrome.

Low dose aspirin is not associated with adverse maternal or fetal outcome. Most interest at present is focused on anti-oxidant vitamin supplementation with vitamin C and vitamin E, which has been associated with a significant reduction in risk of preeclampsia in one randomized controlled trial in high risk women. Although encouraging, this work urgently requires to be repeated on a larger scale. In women with established severe, early onset pre-eclampsia such therapy has not been found to be beneficial.

Mild/moderate PIH

Mild/moderate hypertension is usually picked up as a blood pressure between 90-110mmHg diastolic with no proteinuria at antenatal check. These women should have a repeat BP measurement four hours later. If hypertension is confirmed, basic surveillance of twice weekly monitoring of BP/Urine and clinical assessment of maternal and fetal well being is required. Full blood count, urea and electrolytes and urate should be obtained. Enhanced surveillance is required if, i). the DBP is greater than 100mmHg at gestations less than 37 weeks; ii). the blood pressure increment is greater than 25mmHg; iii). there is clinical suspicion of IUGR; iv). concern over maternal or fetal wellbeing, or v). abnormal biochemistry.

Enhanced surveillance takes the form of thrice weekly assessment of BP, urine and full blood count , urea and electrolytes and urate, and liver function tests. An assessment of the fetus should also be made including fetal growth, cardiotocography (CTG) or biophysical profile[3]. There is no indication for admission or bed rest for these women unless further abnormalities are found such as evidence of fetal compromise or abnormal biochemistry for example deranged liver function tests or significant proteinuria.

Therefore, care can be managed, effectively both clinically and in terms of cost, through a day care unit and/or in the community. The value of antihypertensive therapy is these women is uncertain. Although there may be a reduction in the progression to proteinuric disease and severe hypertension, there is no benefit in terms of gestation at delivery or obstetric intervention. Thus, perhaps antihypertensive therapy should be reserved for early onset disease (<32 wks) or DBP >100mmHg, although the reduction in proteinuria and severe hypertension may be of value in reducing the perceived need for intervention.

While some go on to develop severe disease, many, particularly those with late onset hypertension have a benign course for the remainder of their pregnancy. Blood pressure tends to return to normal within a few weeks postpartum. As these women are at increased risk of chronic hypertension in later life, persistent hypertension 6 weeks after delivery will require investigation.

Severe disease and the fulminating preeclamptic

Severe disease requires admission to hospital for clinical, biochemical, hematological and fetal assessment. As severe disease is often of early onset the key objective is to prolong pregnancy without risk to the mother. An average prolongation of two weeks can be achieved with associated reduction in neonatal morbidity. There is little place for conservative management of women with proteinuric disease at ≥34 weeks gestation.

Magnesium sulphate, is now the prophylactic anticonvulsant of choice for women at risk of eclampsia and will significantly reduce the risk of eclampsia for women with pre-eclampsia. Fulminating preeclampsia, where the woman is symptomatic, with epigastric pain, headache and visual disturbance, or where blood pressure is uncontrolled, or where hematological and biochemical investigations are rapidly deteriorating requires urgent, usually operative, delivery after stabilization with antihypertenasive therapy and magnesium sulphate. Care must be taken to avoid fluid overload, which can be followed by pulmonary edema and/or ARDS which may be fatal. Acute cardiac dysfunction is probably underreported and should be sought with echocardiography. These patients are also at risk of venous thromboembolism and require thromboprophylaxis.

Eclampsia may be arise without warning or may be preceded by the classical prodrome of headache, visual disturbance, and epigastric pain. It may occur for the first time after delivery. Control of seizures with magnesium sulphate and control of blood pressure followed by delivery are the mainstays of treatment.

Following delivery, preeclampsia will resolve although the hypertension and proteinuria may take several weeks to do so. In the immediate postpartum period, preeclampsia may initially worsen.

Long term outcome

Mothers who experience uncomplicated pregnancies have a lower incidence of subsequent hypertension compared with the general population. In contrast pregnancies complicated by early onset disease have an increased in risk of hypertension in later life. Women with a history of pre-eclampsia have higher circulating levels of fasting insulin, lipid and coagulation factors post-partum relative to BMI matched controls and also have an increased risk of coronary artery disease Thus the genotypes and phenotypes underlying vascular disease may also underlie pre-eclampsia[2].

Treatment of hypertension in pregnancy

Treatment of blood pressure in pregnancy is aimed at reducing both maternal and fetal risk of complications. While long term blood pressure reduction outwith pregnancy aims to prevent cerebrovascular and cardiovascular sequelae, mild/moderate hypertension in pregnancy may have a good outcome in the absence of pre-eclampsia. The higher diastolic blood pressure, the greater the benefit of treatment, and treatment of a DBP of 110 mmHg or greater has been shown to reduce the incidence of stroke and cardiovascular complications. While some opt not to treat milder elevations of blood pressure (DBP 90-100 mmHg), treatment may reduce the incidence of premature delivery, frequency of hospitalization, and possibly delay the onset of proteinurias as noted above. Where pre-eclampsia has supervened, the aim of blood pressure management is to provide protection from complications such as stroke, renal impairment, eclampsia, placental abruption and ante-partum hemorrhage until delivery can be expedited.

Choice of therapy

- **Methyldopa**

    When hypertension is present in early pregnancy, methyldopa remains the treatment of choice. Multiple daily dosing and stepwise titration of dosage are necessary. Its central action causes adverse effects such as drowsiness, lethargy and nasal stuffiness. It is known to be safe for the fetus with no residual adverse developmental effects seen up to school age. It is probably best avoided postpartum due to the association with depression

- **ß-blockers**

    There are some concerns that prolonged use of ß-blockers in pregnancy may result in intra-uterine growth restriction, but recent studies suggest that this is phenomenon of antihypertensive therapy in general rather than a specific effect of ß-blockers. Atenolol and labetalol have been shown to be as safe and effective as methyldopa when administered in the third trimester, and may be better tolerated. Intravenous labetalol is useful for the emergency treatment of blood pressure in pre-eclampsia/eclampsia. Intravenous hydralazine or sublingual nifedipine were used in the past, but may cause precipitous falls in blood pressure.

- **Dihydropyridine calcium antagonists (Nifedipine)**

    Nifedipine is not licensed for use in pregnancy but is effective at lowering blood pressure and is favoured as a useful second-line agent in pre-eclampsia, to allow pregnancy to continue in order to permit fetal maturation.

- **Hydralazine**
  Hydralazine, has traditionally been used as a second line agent and intravenously for hypertensive crises. Although effective in reducing blood pressure, labetalol and nifedipine are superior in terms of episodes of maternal hypertension, incidence of abruption, Caesarean section and side effects.

- **Thiazide diuretics**
  Thiazides are not recommended during pregnancy, due to a theoretical risk of exacerbating pre-eclampsia by restricting plasma expansion. While most obstetricians would avoid their use there is evidence that they are effective at attenuating blood pressure rise during pregnancy; thus, low dose diuretic therapy, although not fully evaluated, is probably safe. In women who become pregnant while taking low dose thiazides, therapy may be continued unless pre-eclampsia intervenes. Loop diuretics can be needed in severe eclampsia during or after Caesarean section, to treat heart failure.

- **ACE inhibitors**
  ACE inhibitors are contraindicated in pregnancy and should therefore be used with caution in women of childbearing potential. They may be associated with teratogenesis, and in particular may cause abnormalities of the renal tract. Angiotensin II receptor blockers are untested but probably similar. ACE inhibitors are useful postpartum, particularly in women poorly responsive to methyldopa or labetalol and are not contraindicated in breast-feeding.

Summary
Hypertension per se is not a contraindication to pregnancy. Accurate measurement, pre-pregnancy advice where appropriate, regular follow-up and adequate treatment maximizes the likelihood of a successful outcome. Pre-eclampsia is serious and eclampsia life threatening; both require specialist management.

Oral contraceptives and hormone replacement therapy
The estrogen-containing oral contraceptive pill (OCP) causes a small rise in blood pressure in most women, probably due to renin-angiotensin II – mediated volume expansion. However, only about 5% of users over 5 years will develop hypertension, about three times more than among non-users. The risk of developing hypertension is greatest in women over 35, the obese and in those who drink excess alcohol. Hypertension in a previous pregnancy also increases the risk of subsequent hypertension with oral contraceptives.

Most doctors withdraw estrogen-containing OCP if there is a rise in blood pressure, and try the progestogen-only pill instead. Other physicians prefer to treat any mild hypertension with drug therapy while maintaining estrogen OCP, in patients where pregnancy would be most undesirable for the particular individual. Neither approach is absolutely right for every woman, and patient involvement in decision making is important.

When oral contraceptives are discontinued after hypertension develops, blood pressure falls back to normal over 3-6 months in about half of the women. Among those whose blood pressure remains elevated, it is not known whether the contraceptives precipitated the onset of hypertension that was going to develop later anyway. Low dose estrogens have a lesser hypertensive effect and may be safer.

Estrogens as part of hormone replacement therapy (HRT) in postmenopausal women are given at a low dose which does not cause a rise in blood pressure. HRT protects women from osteoporosis. However, emerging evidence suggests that HRT is not as safe as once thought. It provides no protection from cardiovascular disease and some forms increase the risk of MI, stroke and thromboembolism. HRT also increases the risk of breast cancer, particularly in women with a first degree relative with breast cancer.

HYPERTENSION
Diastolic BP of >/= 110mmHg on any one occasion
OR
Diastolic BP of >/= 90mmHg on any two or more consecutive occasions >/= 4 hours apart.

SEVERE HYPERTENSION
Diastolic BP >/= 120mmHg on any one occasion
OR
Diastolic BP >/= 110mmHg on two or more consecutive occasions >/=4 hours apart.

PROTEINURIA
One 24-hour urine collection with a total protein excretion of >/= 300mg/24hrs.
OR
Two midstream or catheter specimens of urine (collected >/=4 hours apart) with >/= "++" protein on reagent strip testing.
OR
3 "+" protein (If Urine SG <1.030 AND pH </= 8)

Table 1. Classification of hypertension in pregnancy.

Positive risk factors	Negative risk Factors
Positive risk factors First pregnancy to a partner (ie primipaternity) Previous pre-eclampsia Central obesity Migraine Age <20 and >35 years Maternal family history of pre-eclampsia Diabetes Congenital and acquired thrombophilia Renal and connective tissue disease Essential hypertension Multiple pregnancy Hydrops and molar pregnancy Fetal trisomy	Previous pregnancy reaching the second trimester and not complicated by pre-eclampsia Long period of sexual cohabitation Smoking

Table 2. Risk factors for pre-eclampsia.

References

1. Greer, I.A. (2001). Pregnancy-induced hypertension. In: (Ed. Chamberlain G.V.P. & Steer, P.J.). Turnbull's Obstetrics 3d Edition Chuchill Livingstone, London. pp 333 – 353.

2. Sattar, N & Greer, I.A. (2002). Pregnancy complications and maternal cardiovascular risk : opportunities for intervention and screening? British Medical Journal 325,157-60.

3. SOGAP 1997 The Management of mild, non-proteinuric hypertension in pregnancy. A clinical practice guideline for professionals involved in maternity care in Scotland. Scottish Obstetric Guidelines and Audit Project. Scottish Programme for Clinical Effectiveness in Reproductive Health

CHAPTER 12

HYPERTENSION: SPECIAL ISSUES IN DIFFERENT ETHNIC GROUPS

Neil Chapman, Jamil Mayet and Adrian Brady

Introduction

There are two main ethnic minorities in the UK, namely African-Caribbeans and South Asians (those from the Indian sub-continent). Although African-Caribbeans constitute a genetically diverse group, they have many characteristics in common and will be considered in this chapter as a single group.

Compared with Caucasians, both hypertension and its complications are more common in both main ethnic minorities. Possible differences in etiology, frequency of co-morbid conditions and response to treatment mean that the ethnic origin of a hypertensive patient must be considered in their management.

Prevalence of hypertension and its complications

Hypertension is more prevalent among patients from ethnic minorities than among UK Caucasians. Compared with Caucasians, in a recent community-based study in South London, high blood pressure (BP) was 2.6 times as common in African-Caribbeans and 1.8 times as common in South Asians.[1] Average BP varies between different sub-groups of South Asians, being highest in Sikhs, similar to Caucasians in Muslims and intermediate in Hindus.[2]

In addition, patterns of hypertension-associated morbidity and mortality vary between different ethnic groups. Relative to Caucasians, mortality from ischemic heart disease is more common in South Asians but less common in African-Caribbeans (Figure 1a). African-Caribbeans, however, have a high incidence of congestive heart failure. Mortality from stroke (Figure 1b) and the incidence of end-stage renal failure are more common in both ethnic groups, particularly African-Caribbeans.[3]

The reasons for differences in prevalence of hypertension and its associated morbidity and mortality are still not fully understood. Although there is undoubtedly some confounding effect of social class, differences probably reflect complex interactions between genetics, other environmental factors and co-existing cardiovascular risk factors.

Secular trends in hypertension in ethnic minorities

The pattern of hypertension-associated morbidity and mortality is changing (Figure 1). Excess African-Caribbean mortality from stroke declined sharply between 1970-2 and 1989-92. This may reflect an improvement in socio-economic status but is also likely to be due to an increased awareness of the problem among patients and their medical practitioners. Indeed, a recent study found that African-Caribbean hypertensives were more likely to have been diagnosed than either South Asians or Caucasians.[1]

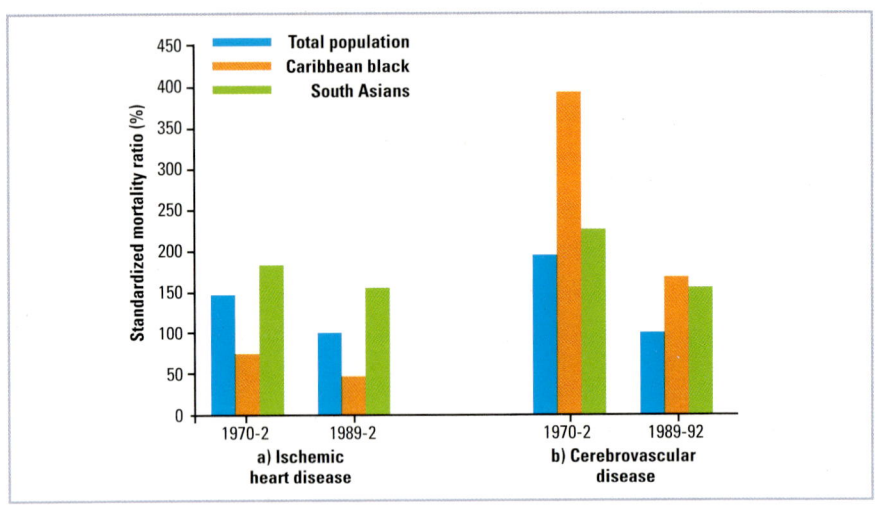

Figure 1. *Standardized mortality ratios (SMR) for (a) Ischemic heart disease (IHD) and (b) cerebrovascular disease in the total population, Caribbean Blacks and South Asians in the years 1970-2 and 1989-92. The reference value of 100 is deaths from either IHD or cerebrovascular disease in the total population in the 1989-92 period. (Adapted from Wild and McKeigue, 1997.)*

Mechanisms of hypertension in ethnic minorities

Most work on ethnic differences in hypertension has compared Caucasians with African-Caribbeans living in the United States. Although BP is relatively low in certain rural African communities, urbanized Africans and those who have emigrated tend to have higher BP than Caucasians. Such alterations, demonstrated in migration studies, may parallel changes in dietary content. In the West, differences between BP in African-Caribbeans and Caucasians are usually apparent from childhood.[3]

African-Caribbeans have enhanced sensitivity to sodium, reduced renal sodium excretion and a less reactive renin-angiotensin-aldosterone system. Low serum potassium occurs more frequently in African-Caribbeans than in Caucasians in the absence of diuretic therapy or hyperaldosteronism. Relative to Caucasians, African-Caribbeans tend to have a higher peripheral resistance and a lower cardiac output. Furthermore, African-Caribbeans exhibit a smaller degree of nocturnal BP dip than Caucasians (Figure 2) and their higher night-time BP may partly explain an increased prevalence of left ventricular hypertrophy.

Prevalence of co-existing cardiovascular risk factors

Ethnic differences in patterns of morbidity and mortality may partly be explained by differences in other cardiovascular risk factors (Figure 3). Obesity and diabetes are both common in ethnic minority patients, with a particularly high prevalence among African-Caribbean females.[1]

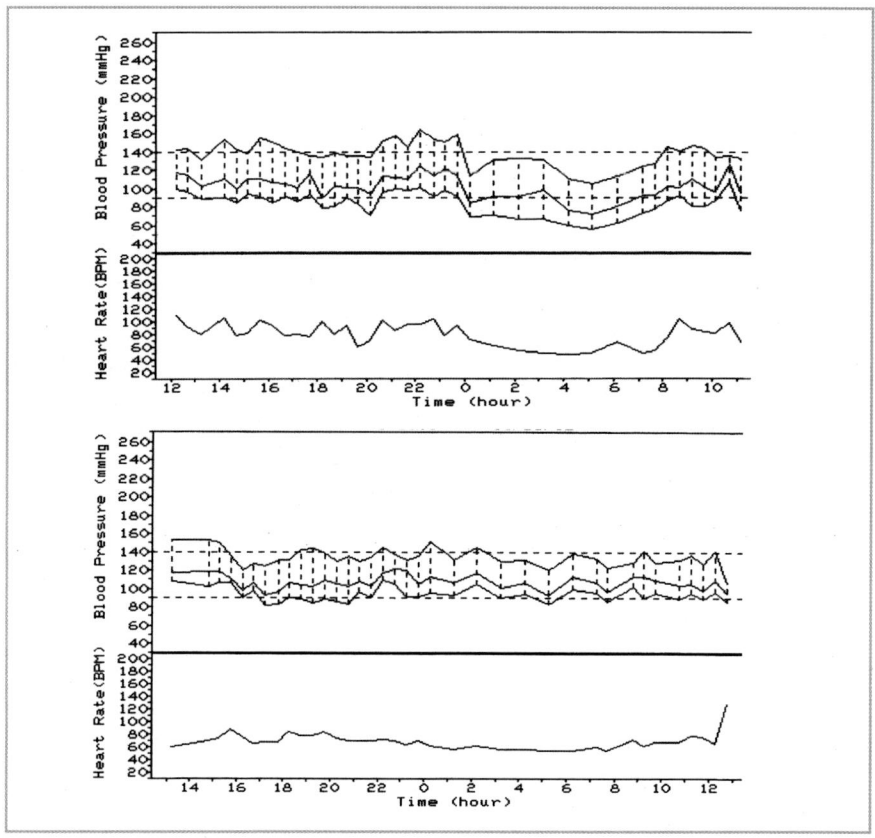

Figure 2. Examples of 24 hour ambulatory blood pressure monitoring showing a profile from a Caucasian subject (top) with a normal nocturnal BP dip and a profile from an African-Caribbean subject (bottom) with attenuation of the nocturnal dip.

Left ventricular hypertrophy (LVH) is associated with hypertension, but is a more powerful independent predictor of cardiovascular morbidity and mortality than high BP itself. LVH is more common in African-Caribbeans than in other ethnic groups and this may help to explain the excess incidence of sudden death and prevalence of congestive heart failure in this group. However, ethnic differences in prevalence of LVH may be exaggerated when diagnosed using ECG rather than echocardiography: voltages generated by a given myocardial mass appear to be larger in African-Caribbeans compared with Caucasians.

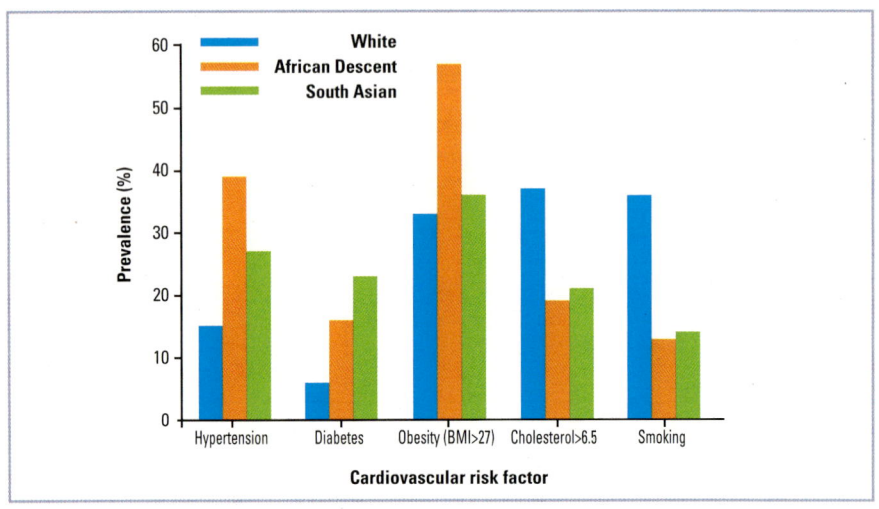

Figure 3: Age-adjusted prevalence of cardiovascular disease risk factors in Whites, those of African descent and South Asians. Hypertension was defined as systolic BP ≥ 160 and/or diastolic BP ≥ 95 mmHg, or on anti-hypertensive drug treatment.
Diabetes was defined according to WHO criteria. BMI, body mass index (kg/m2).
(Adapted from Cappuccio et al, 1997).

The high incidence of ischemic heart disease in South Asians may be explained, at least in part, by the high prevalence of the insulin resistance syndrome 2 as defined to include central obesity, type 2 diabetes and dyslipidemia (high plasma triglycerides and low HDL-cholesterol), in addition to hypertension. Identification and education of hypertensive patients from ethnic minorities.

Awareness of the high prevalence of hypertension in ethnic minority groups should direct medical practitioners towards especially careful screening in patients from these groups. If targets for the control of BP are to be achieved, education about the risks of hypertension and the benefits of treatment is vital, and may improve patient compliance. It has been suggested that poor compliance is a factor in the relatively high mortality rates among African-Caribbeans, although there is little evidence for this. Where necessary, education should involve an appropriate interpreter and should stress the importance of both non-pharmacological and drug treatment.

Non-pharmacological management

Non-pharmacological measures can be an effective means of lowering both blood pressure and associated cardiovascular risk. As both African-Caribbeans and South Asians are more likely to be overweight, dietary advice on restriction of calorie intake is important. This advice should be tailored to an individual patient's ethnic group and existing dietary habit, and where necessary, should be available in the patient's own language.

African-Caribbeans often eat a diet low in potassium and high in sodium. As they are particularly sodium-sensitive, moderate restriction of dietary sodium and an increase in dietary potassium may have a particularly beneficial effect on BP. In addition, salt restriction, by activation of the renin-angiotensin axis, may improve responsiveness to anti-hypertensive drugs acting on this system.[3]

In South Asians, restriction of dietary saturated fat combined with weight loss and regular aerobic exercise improves the metabolic abnormalities of the insulin resistance syndrome and reduces overall cardiovascular risk.[2]

Pharmacological treatment

From the limited evidence available, South Asians appear to respond to anti-hypertensive drug therapy in a similar manner to Caucasians. The most effective drugs, and therefore the drugs of choice in an otherwise uncomplicated African-Caribbean hypertensive, are diuretics or calcium-channel blockers. In terms of BP reduction, both are as effective, if not more so, than in Caucasians (Figure 4). Due to a less reactive renin-angiotensin axis, African-Caribbeans usually respond poorly to monotherapy with ACE inhibitors and ß-blockers, which depend for their action either mainly or partly on inhibiting activation of this system. This deficiency may be overcome by the addition of a low-dose diuretic, such as a thiazide.[3]

It has been suggested that the presence of cardiovascular structural or metabolic abnormalities associated with hypertension may influence the initial choice of anti-hypertensive drug. ACE-inhibitors appear to be the most effective drugs in causing regression of LVH, and may have effects beyond those of BP lowering. Thus in an African-Caribbean with LVH, an ACE-inhibitor, possibly in combination with a low-dose thiazide diuretic, may be the drug of choice. Similarly, African-Caribbean patients with ischemic heart disease may benefit from a beta-blocking agent, with or without additional anti-hypertensives.

Overall, there do appear to be ethnic differences in the efficacy of anti-hypertensive drugs. Cases in which the preferred drug might be expected to be less effective can be overcome using appropriate non-pharmacological or drug measures. Therefore, where co-existing disease or target-organ damage dictates the choice of anti-hypertensive agent, ethnic origin should not deter the physician from prescribing the appropriate drug.

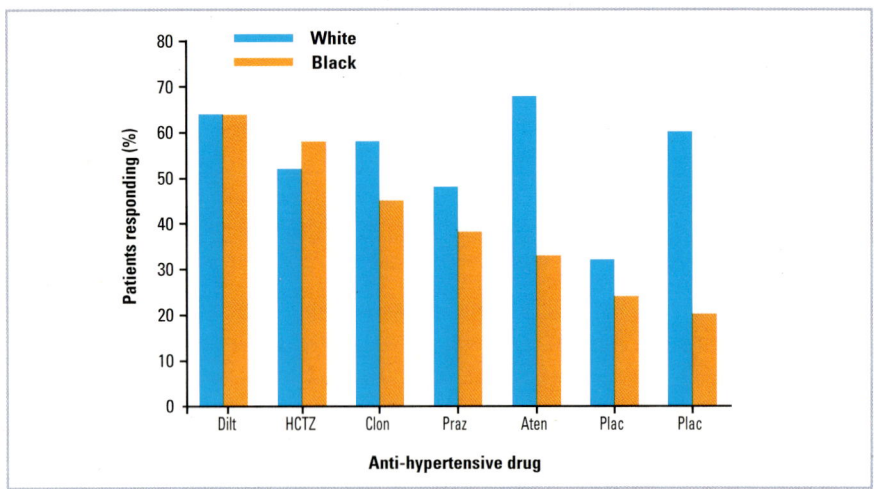

Figure 4: Percentage of White and African-Caribbean hypertensive patients (≥ 60 years) responding to anti-hypertensive monotherapy. Response to therapy defined as diastolic BP < 90mmHg at the end of 4-8 week titration period and < 95 mmHg after 1 year of treatment. Dilt, Diltiazem; HCTZ, Hydrochlorothiazide; Clon, Clonidine; Praz, Prazosin; Aten, Atenolol; Plac, Placebo; Capt, Captopril. (Adapted from Materson et al, 1993).

Summary

Differences exist between ethnic groups in the UK with regard to the prevalence, likely etiology and response to treatment of hypertension. Differences also exist in co-existing diseases, which may influence cardiovascular morbidity and mortality. The assessment, investigation and management, both non-pharmacological and pharmacological, of people with hypertension must therefore consider ethnic origin.

Key Points

● Hypertension is more common among ethnic minorities in the UK than in Caucasians

● Patterns of cardiovascular disease and mortality differ between ethnic groups and may reflect differences in co-existing diseases and risk factors

● Response to anti-hypertensive drugs varies between ethnic groups, particularly between Caucasians and African-Caribbeans

References

1. Cappuccio FP, Cook DG, Atkinson RW, Strazzullo P. Prevalence, detection, and management of cardiovascular risk factors in different ethnic groups in South London. *Heart* 1997; 78: 555-563.

2. McKeigue PM, Shah B, Marmot MG. Relation of central obesity and insulin resistance with high diabetes prevalence and cardiovascular risk in South Asians. *Lancet* 1991; 337: 382-386.

3. Kaplan NM. Ethnic aspects of hypertension. *Lancet* 1994; 344: 450-2.

CHAPTER 13

HYPERTENSION AND ENDOCRINE DISEASE
Stephen Cleland and Adrian Brady

Introduction

Hypertension is a feature of a number of endocrine disorders, including acromegaly, Cushing's syndrome and thyroid disease. It can be the presenting feature of an endocrine condition such as pheochromocytoma. Overall, endocrine causes of high blood pressure are relatively rare (estimates vary from 1-3%).

The importance of endocrine causes of hypertension is two-fold. First, the identification of an endocrine cause of hypertension often leads to cure of high blood pressure; in some instances a life-threatening disorder, such as phaeochromocytoma may be corrected. Secondly, the study of endocrine forms of hypertension has elucidated important aspects of endocrine physiology and pathophysiology. In this brief review we will consider the major forms of endocrine hypertension encountered in clinical practice.

Corticosteroids and hypertension[1]

I. Glucocorticoids

Glucocorticoid excess causes hypertension in humans and in experimental animals (see Ref 2 for review). In man, the principal glucocorticoid is cortisol, acting at specific receptors in a wide range of target tissues. Cortisol excess due to Cushing's syndrome is associated with hypertension in over 50% of cases (Fig 1). This is also a feature of iatrogenic glucocorticoid excess using synthetic hormones such as prednisolone and dexamethasone.

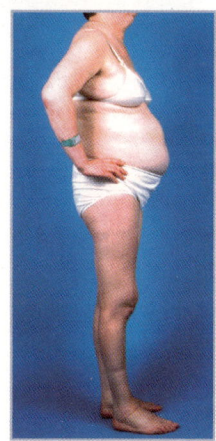

The cause of glucocorticoid-induced hypertension remains uncertain. Cortisol excess causes acute renal sodium retention, but long term glucocorticoid hypertension (e.g. Cushing's syndrome) is not typically associated with either suppression of plasma renin or hypokalaemia, both of which would be expected to be found in sodium-dependent forms of

Figure 1. photograph of patient with Cushing's Syndrome

130

hypertension (ectopic ACTH syndrome is an exception, where hypokalemia is often found). Studies in experimental animals and in humans have indicated that acute and chronic glucocorticoid excess also alters vasodilator prostanoid synthesis, increases pressor sensitivity to alpha-adrenoreceptor stimulation and, possibly, most importantly, alters vascular endothelial nitric oxide production. Thus, there are likely to be a range of mechanisms which result in glucocorticoid hypertension in humans. Depending on the reason for cortisol excess, surgery may be a treatment option - for example, removal of an ACTH-secreting pituitary microadenoma or adrenalectomy. If patients are unsuitable for surgery, medical treatment with drugs such as metyrapone is an option, although side-effects with such agents may be a problem.

II. Mineralocorticoid hypertension

Mineralocorticoid hypertension is, typically, associated with renal sodium retention, potassium wasting (with consequent hypokalaemia if this becomes excessive) and suppression of plasma renin activity. The classical form of mineralocorticoid hypertension is exemplified by primary aldosteronism, most commonly due to an adrenal adenoma secreting aldosterone (Conn's syndrome). These benign tumours, which are generally small, produce aldosterone independent of regulation by renin (fig 2).

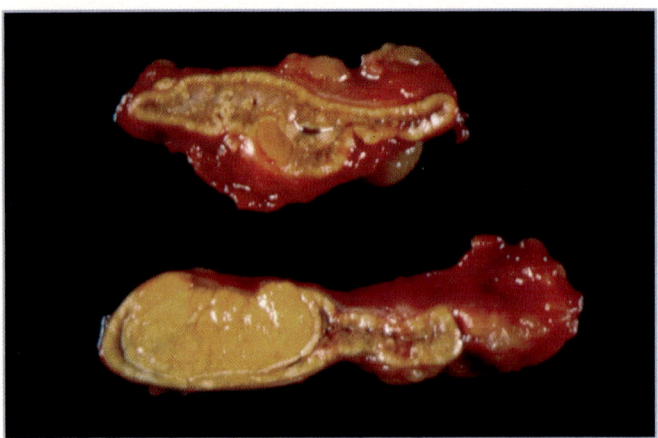

Figure 2. Aldosterone-secreting adrenal adenoma, removed after curative surgery for Conn's syndrome

As a consequence, patients exhibit suppression of plasma renin, with aldosterone values which are either at the upper end of the normal range or frankly elevated. Initially, Conn's syndrome was thought to be a relatively rare cause of hypertension, accounting for less than 1% of cases. More recently, however, studies using a sensitive renin-angiotensin ratio as a screening test, have suggested that primary aldosteronism due to Conn's syndrome is relatively common, and some claims suggest that it may be found in as many as 10% of patients with high blood pressure.[3] This screening test may be useful in clinical practice, and can be used in patients taking anti-hypertensive medication. However, it should be interpreted in the context of other features including more detailed dynamic tests and appropriate imaging investigations.

Primary aldosteronism can also be found in patients without a localizing adenoma, when the condition is due to bilateral adrenal hyperplasia. Clearly, distinguishing these patients from those with a solitary adenoma is important, as in these circumstances adrenal surgery is inappropriate.

For this reason, in the absence of a clearly identified unilateral lesion on adrenal CT scanning, adrenal vein sampling for measurement of aldosterone can help localize hormone production and, consequently, guide the need for surgical therapy. In the absence of surgical treatment therapy with either amiloride or spironolactone is often effective in controlling hypertension.

More rarely, mineralocorticoid-type hypertension can occur in a number of genetic forms. These include glucocorticoid-suppressible hyperaldosteronism, apparent mineralocorticoid excess, Liddle's syndrome and inborn errors of adrenal steroid metabolism.

Pheochromocytoma

Tumors of the adrenal medulla are a rare, but eminently curable form of endocrine hypertension.[4] The incidence of pheochromocytoma is rare, accounting for < 0.1% of patients with high blood pressure. These tumors are usually found in the adrenal medulla, but also occur in other neurone ectoderm-derived tissue. Most phechromocytomas (90%) are benign tumors but a small number (10%) are malignant and these may metastasize to liver and bone.

About 10% of pheochromocytomas occur outside the adrenal, generally within the abdomen. Patients may present with a classical history of paroxysmal symptoms, such as palpitation, sweating and acute anxiety, but the diagnosis should be considered in other circumstances: for example, hypertension resistant to conventional agents, marked variability in blood pressure readings, or hypertension where control deteriorates after ß-blockade, because of unopposed α-adrenoceptor activity.

The majority of pheochromocytomas secrete noradrenaline, although a small percentage predominantly produce adrenaline. In addition, a number of other peptide hormones with pressor activity can be produced by these tumors, including neuropeptide Y and endothelin.

Diagnosis of pheochromocytoma is most easily made by measurement of catecholamines or catecholamine metabolites in 24-hour urine collections or by plasma catecholamines. In a small number of patients, however, production of hormones by tumors may be paroxysmal and several collections may be necessary where diagnostic suspicion is high. In some circumstances a clonidine suppression test may help differentiate between borderline noradrenaline excess of neural origin and that due to a pheochromocytoma.

Localization of pheochromocytoma may be carried out by using MRI scanning (Fig 3). In situations in which there is no obvious adrenal tumor, imaging with metaiobenzylguanidine (MIBG) may be helpful. Occasionally, venous sampling may be required to provide more accurate localization, particularly for tumors lying outside the abdomen. The old fashioned description of the "10% tumor": 10% are multiple; 10% are familial; 10% are bilateral and 10% are malignant, is roughly true.

Some pheochromocytomas are familial, and the majority of these tumors are bilateral. It is important, therefore, to take an accurate family history in patients with this disorder. In addition, patients with a familial history may have multiple endocrine neoplasia type II syndrome (MEN IIA) which includes medullary carcinoma of the thyroid and parathyroid hyperplasia.

This autosomal dominant condition, now recognized to be due to an abnormality on chromosome 10 is generally associated with bilateral pheochromocytomas. For this reason it is mandatory that the diagnosis of MEN IIA is considered in all patients presenting with phaeochromocytoma, and that their plasma calcitonin is measured. Conversely, all patients presenting with medullary carcinoma of the thyroid need screening for pheochromocytoma. Long term follow-up of these patients is essential,

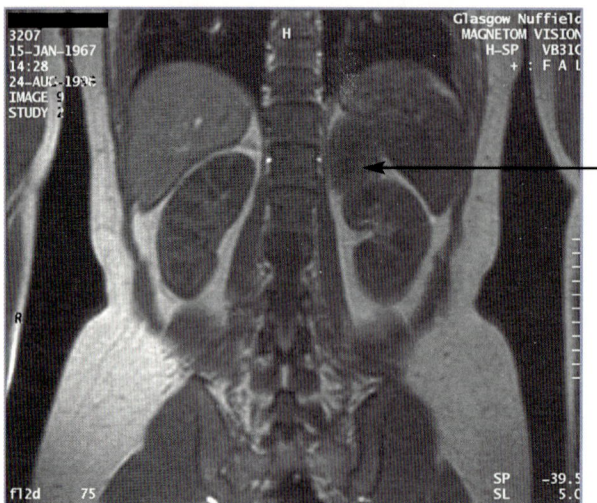

pheochromocytoma

Figure 3.

as is detailed family screening; which has now been simplified by the availability of appropriate genetic markers.

The treatment of choice is surgical removal of the tumor. Pre-operative treatment with an α-blocker (phenoxybenzamine) is essential, and ß₁-blocker therapy may also be used to deal with tachycardia. It is important to ensure adequate α-blockade prior to ß-blocker therapy because unopposed ß-blockade in patients with pheochromocytoma.

Acromegaly
Growth hormone (GH) excess has adverse effects on the cardiovascular system, most notably in the form of hypertension and left ventricular hypertrophy, and later, cardiomyopathy. The latter can be a feature of acromegaly in the absence of hypertension and, therefore, is likely to be secondary to trophic effects of GH, possibly mediated by insulin-like growth factor-1 (IGF-1).

The precise mechanism of hypertension in acromegaly remains unknown. Total exchangeable sodium is increased in this condition, which suggests that the hypertension may be sodium-dependent. In support of this view, plasma renin activity tends to be reduced in acromegaly. Mineralocorticoid excess is not a feature of acromegaly, suggesting that sodium retention is due to either a direct action of GH/IGF-1 on renal tubules or to a blunting of the physiological secretion of atrial natriuretic peptide.

It has also been suggested that changes in sympathetic nerve activity may be responsible for hypertension in acromegaly, but the evidence for this is conflicting. Removal of excess GH can result in normalization of blood pressure, but in some cases hypertension persists and should be treated with conventional therapy (see Ref 5 for review).

Thyroid disease
Hypertension is reportedly associated with both hyper- and hypothyroidism.[5] Thyrotoxicosis is usually associated with a high cardiac output, tachycardia including atrial arrhythmias, peripheral vasodilatation and systolic hypertension, which resolve after normalization of thyroid status. Hypothyroidism may be associated with diastolic hypertension which tends to resolve following thyroid replacement, although few well controlled studies have adequately taken into account placebo effects and the tendency for blood pressure to fall with repeated measurements. The mechanism of "hypothyroid hypertension" is unknown, but may involve sodium and water retention or possible changes in sensitivity to circulating catecholamines. If hypertension persists several months after normalization of thyroid status, conventional anti-hypertensive therapy should be instituted.

Hyperparathyroidism
Hypertension is reported to be associated with hyperparathyroidism in 10-60% of cases.[6] Surgical removal of the parathyroid adenoma usually causes normalization of blood pressure. Parathyroid hormone itself may directly raise blood pressure, but there is also

evidence for the existence of co-secreted plasma factor which may be responsible for the hypertension in this condition. An increased calcium concentration, for whatever reason, may be involved in abnormal vascular smooth muscle control resulting in hypertension. However, the data on calcium levels and blood pressure are unclear and often contradictory. As with thyroid disease, there are relatively few well controlled studies on blood pressure regulation in relation to parathyroid disease. Again, hypertension that persists after normalization of parathyroid status should be tackled by conventional means. Secondary hyperparathyroidism from chronic renal failure can occur, and these patients are usually hypertensive from their renal condition.

Keypoints

- Underlying endocrine disorders may account for 1-3% of hypertension.

- Endogenous glucocorticoid excess can cause hypertension and may be amenable to surgical treatment.

- Mineralocorticoid hypertension due to Conn's Syndrome may be more prevalent than previously thought.

- Pheochromocytoma may present in association with other potentially life threatening endocrine disorders.

- Acromegaly, hyperthyroidism, hypothyroidism and hyperparathyroidism can cause hypertension; however, high blood pressure may persist despite normalization of hormone levels.

References

1. Fraser R, Davies DL, Connell JMC. Hormones and hypertension. *Clin Endocrin* 1989; 31: 701-746.

2. Fraser R, Connell JMC. Corticosteroids and hypertension. *J Hypertension* 1991; 7: 97-107.

3. Gordon RD, Zlesak MD, Tunney TT et al. Evidence that primary aldosteronism may not be uncommon: 12% incidence among antihypertensive drug trial volunteers. *Clin Exp Pharmacol Physiol* 1993; 20: 296-298.

4. Ross EJ, Griffith DNW. The clinical presentation of phaeochromocytoma. Q J Med 1989; 71:485-496.

5. Streeten DHP, Anderson GH, Howland T, Chiang R, Smulyan H. Effect of thyroid function on blood pressure - recognition of hypothyroid hypertension. *Hypertension* 1988; 11: 78-83.

6. Sangal AV, Beevers DG. Parathyroid hypertension. *Bri Med J* 1983; 286: 498-499.

CHAPTER 14

HYPERTENSION AND STROKE Pankaj Sharma, Adrian Brady, Kennedy Lees

Acute stroke has an incidence rate approximately 380 per 100,000. It remains the third biggest killer in the West, and a non-fatal stroke is often a devastating blow to an individual. Stroke is a clinically defined syndrome causing focal neurological symptoms which last greater than 24 hours. The distinction from a transient ischemic attack (TIA) is arbitrary and now criticized.

This simple definition of stroke, however, belies the complexity and heterogeneous nature of a condition which can vary clinically from a clouding of vision to deep coma, and range pathologically from a hemorrhage to small vessel disease, ischemia or emboli. Indeed, it is partly this heterogeneity that has contributed to the slow progress of specific therapy, stroke remaining perhaps two decades behind myocardial infarction. However, with technological advances in imaging and developments in thrombolysis the situation is changing.

Diagnosis and examination of acute stroke
The history and clinical features of a sudden (indicating a vascular) event causing a focal neurological deficit should be enough to make the diagnosis of a stroke. An additional history of risk factors such as previous TIA, myocardial infarction, atrial fibrillation or other arrhythmia, hypertension or smoking is often encountered. A family history is occasionally found in younger patients with a stroke while a history of trauma (particularly to the neck), contraceptive pill use or illicit drug use may suggest less common causes of a stroke.

Targeting drug therapy in the acute stroke victim
Investigators seeking new drugs to treat stroke have targeted events during the early hours after stroke onset. Final development of cerebral infarction takes several hours (and possibly longer) to establish itself once injury has commenced. The eventual infarct volume comprises an early central necrotic zone surrounded by a poorly perfused penumbral region. As morbidity is directly related to the site and size of the infarct it is therefore this potentially viable and reversible ischemic penumbra where drug development has concentrated. Although the penumbra may be viable for several hours, in practice drugs need to act within a very short window of opportunity.

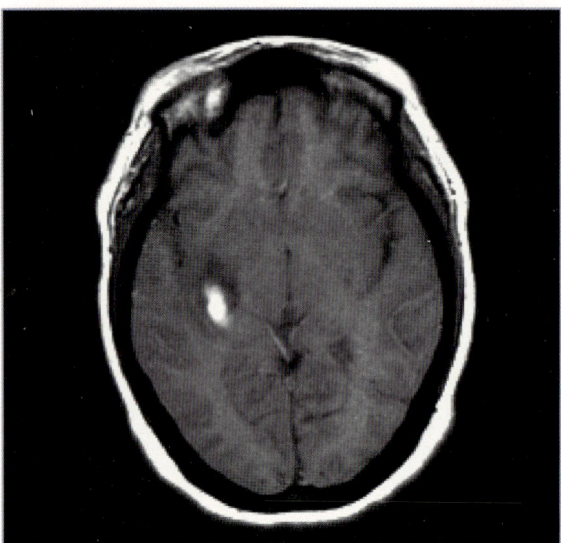

Figure 1. MRI of intracranial hemorrhage.

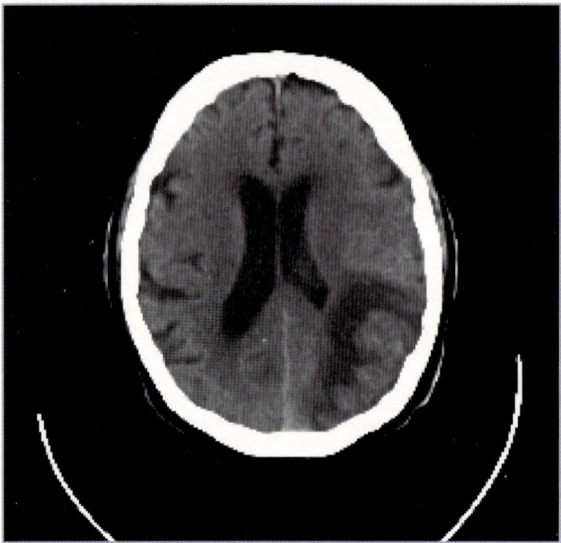

Figure 2. Left occipital infarct with surrounding edema.

Thrombolytic therapy

The 1995 NINDS (National Institute of Neurological Disorders and Stroke) trial demonstrated that thrombolysis with rt-PA within three hours of stroke onset resulted in an 11-13% absolute increase in the proportion of patients who made an excellent recovery. Although the treated groups had a rate of intracerebral hemorrhage of 6.4% versus 0.6% in the untreated group with an increase in morbidity at 36 hours, there was no difference in mortality at 3 months, partly reflecting the fact that complications are greatest in patients with the largest strokes. Stroke thrombolysis is therefore high risk for high gain. The logistics of administering treatment within three hours of stroke onset have limited uptake of this treatment even in the USA, though the most active centres now treat 10-15% of their patients. A European licence for rt-PA within three hours of stroke was recently granted, with encouragement of post-marketing surveillance.

Other thrombolytics have also undergone clinical trials. Streptokinase was extensively investigated but abandoned because of high bleeding risk. Intra-arterial thrombolysis may be beneficial within six hours of stroke but carries greater practical difficulties. Several trials involving other thombolytic drugs in acute stroke either intravenously or intra-arterially are currently in progress, with especial interest when used alongside diffusion MR imaging to select patients with evidence of persisting at-risk but viable tissue.

Antiplatelet therapy

Prophylactic aspirin reduces the risk of ischemic stroke in those deemed to be at-risk. However, its use during an acute attack is more tenuous. Combined results from large trials (International Stroke Trial and the Chinese Acute Stroke Trial) have shown slight reduction in eventual mortality or non-fatal recurrent stroke of a modest nine patients per 1000 treated. It should be routinely given to patients in whom intracerebral hemorrhage has been excluded by imaging.

Heparin

Systematic reviews have so far failed to show clear benefit from any form of heparin in acute stroke. Despite the lack of evidence, intravenous heparin is still widely used in selected cases. Many specialists would prescribe heparin in those with cardioembolic infarction, stroke-in-evolution or vertebrobasilar thrombosis. The risk of hemorrhagic conversion of infarcted tissue is significant, but directly related to the volume of infarcted tissue. Thus, a CT scan prior to treatment is essential to exclude existing hemorrhage, to judge the volume of infarction and to confirm the age of the infarct (since the risk of hemorrhage is probably greatest 24-96 hours after the ischemic insult).

Early Medical Management of The Stroke Victim

Recent studies in the UK have shown that careful optimization of oxygenation, blood glucose, temperature and other simple measures of attentive good care, including early intensive physiotherapy can make substantial and important differences in the recovery of individuals after stroke.

Blood Pressure

BP often rises markedly following cerebral infarction. Until recently it has been believed that this should not be treated as it is most likely a normal homeostatic response. Raised BP may help perfuse the penumbra and thus limit the eventual infarct size. This dogma is now being challenged with at least two ongoing trials of acute blood pressure lowering shortly after the individual is hospitalized. In presence of thrombolysis, blood pressure should not be allowed to rise above 185/110 mmHg.

Dangerously raised BP (e.g. SBP>230 mmHg or DBP> 140 mm Hg) should be treated cautiously with labetalol or nitroprusside. The high BP post-stroke tends to fall over the next few days, reaching its usual level by about day 3. It is important to remember that raised BP following a stroke admission may indicate pre-existing hypertension; in-itself a major cause of stroke. Clearly, for these patients evidence of secondary end-organ damage should be sought.

Recently, a German group has examined the possibility of careful blood pressure lowering in the setting of acute stroke, the ACCESS study. In this study of 342 patients the ARB Candesartan or placebo was used within 72 hours of onset of stroke symptoms in patients with blood pressure >200/110 mm Hg. The combined endpoint of total mortality, cerebral complications and cardiovascular complications was reduced by almost 50% for patients treated with Candesartan initiated within 72 hrs. This intriguing trial will be published in 2003. If this is confirmed in larger studies the acute management of stroke will change substantially.

Some clinicians still actively increase the BP of those few stroke victims whose admission BP is unusually low. This may be justified in the presence of watershed infarction, especially if there is fluctuation of symptoms.

Glucose

Glucose levels should be maintained around the normal range in patients presenting with ischemic stroke. Accumulating evidence suggests that hyperglycemia worsens outcome while hypoglycemia may extend the size of an infarct. The evidence for tight glucose control in diabetics with acute MI is now clear, and this may be the same for acute stroke but trials are in progress.

Temperature

Pyrexia is common following a stroke and is likely to worsen both morbidity and mortality in patients with cerebral infarction. It is unclear whether the cause of the fever is neurogenic in origin but it is certainly true that stroke patients may develop a pyrexia even without superimposed infection. Such pyrexia can and should be treated with antipyretics, e.g., paracetamol. Finally, it is important to remember that immobile patients are prone to respiratory and urinary tract infections and these should be sought and treated appropriately.

Stroke Units

Specialized stroke units save lives. Stroke patients should be moved, or ideally admitted to, such multidisciplinary units as soon as possible. These units are cost effective; the number needed to treat (NNT) to prevent one patient entering long term care is approximately 10 patients and the NNT to allow one to regain independence is between 10-25. The exact mechanism for this improvement is not clear but may be a reflection of avoidance or early recognition of complications including robust treatment of physiological deviations.

Long-term medical management of the stroke victim

Risk factors should be assessed not only in the patient but also in their immediate family as there is some evidence that both risk factors and stroke itself may have an inherited component. Patients who survive a stroke most commonly die eventually of coronary heart disease. The long-term medical management of the stroke victim should involve secondary prevention targeted at all vascular disease. Simply, this means antithrombotic treatment for all ischemic stroke patients, plus antihypertensives and a statin.

Aspirin is the first choice antiplatelet drug and can commence as soon as the CT scan has excluded hemorrhage. The additional of dipyridamole after a week or two if it can be tolerated confers additional benefit; clopidogrel is an alternative to aspirin with marginally greater efficacy and trials are presently testing whether combination with aspirin is safe and effective. Anticoagulation should be considered for those in atrial fibrillation: either immediately if the ischemic damage was very minor or after two to three weeks in larger infarcts.

Blood pressure should be gradually normalized, after the first few days have elapsed; the PROGRESS trial has told us that even 'normotensive' levels are too high and that an ACE inhibitor/diuretic combination can safely be added in most patients (PROGRESS used perindopril 4 mg and indapamide 2-2.5mg).

The PROGRESS trial demonstrated the substantial benefit of lowering elevated blood pressure in survivors of stroke, with fewer further strokes and myocardial events. These benefits occurred in both hypertensive and normotensive individuals. This important study has given confidence to physicians considering treating elevated blood pressure in patients recovering from stroke or major TIA. Use of this drug combination in truly normotensive patients has yet to gain widespread acceptance pending a forthcoming licensing decision.

Furthermore, it is now clear that control of raised blood pressure in diabetics is even more important than control of blood glucose, to prevent stroke and also heart failure. While these data apply mainly to primary prevention, they may be important in secondary prevention also.

Similarly, the Heart Protection Study has suggested that irrespective of cholesterol level, a statin at high dose may further reduce major vascular events (HPS used simvastatin 40 mg). This is especially interesting since in the past there has been a lack of association between stroke and moderately raised cholesterol if ischemic and hemorrhagic stroke were not distinguished. Other large primary and secondary prevention trials of statins in patients at risk of stroke are shortly due to report.

It may be inappropriate simultaneously to recommence pre-existing antihypertensive drugs and to start all of these additional drugs. Side effects can be difficult to attribute (and can be common with dipyridamole). A sensible approach may be to add treatment in stages over the 2-4 weeks from stroke onset. Life-style changes such as stopping smoking (a relative risk of 1.5 for stroke, but much greater for myocardial infarction), increasing exercise and generally reducing obesity should be encouraged. Social deprivation which is associated with an increase in stroke mortality is less easily overcome.

Conclusion

Suffering a stroke has devastating consequences not only on the patient but also on their relatives. As such, no opportunity of reducing its incidence should be missed. Clearly, there are now many approaches to prevent and treat stroke. We believe that while reducing coronary heart disease is important, the single most important reason that we as physicians treat hypertension is to reduce the incidence of stroke.

References

1. Butcher HC et al Ann Int Med 1998.

2. Stroke Lancet 1998; 352; (Suppl 111) 1-30.

3. Stroke. A practical guide to management. Eds. Warlow, Dennis, van Gijn, Hankey, Sandercock, Bamford, Wardlaw. 1996 Oxford. Pub: Blackwell Science.

4. PROGRESS Collaborative Group. Randomised trial of a perindopril-based blood pressure lowering regimen among 6,105 patients with prior stroke or transient ischemic attack. The Lancet 358:1033-1041, 2001.

CHAPTER 15

HYPERTENSION AND ANGINA, AORTIC AND VASCULAR DISEASE *Adrian Brady*

Introduction

The reasons we treat hypertension are to reduce an individual's risk of stroke, coronary heart disease and heart failure, aortic and peripheral vascular disease, renal failure and retinopathy. However, hypertension is often occult among patients until they present with symptoms of angina or vascular disease. This chapter aims to provide guidance for the treatment of high blood pressure among individuals with overt, established coronary heart disease, aortic disease and peripheral vascular disease.

Hypertension and Angina

Most of the major hypertension trials include patients with existing coronary heart disease. For example, in the recent LIFE trial, 16% of the 9193 patients had pre-existing coronary disease. In the HOPE trial the majority of the 9000+ patients had existing coronary heart disease. The reduction in cardiovascular events was similar in both patients with and without pre-existing coronary heart disease.

However, comparing results of blood pressure lowering versus lipid lowering in patients with established coronary disease, treating blood pressure reduces the risk for further myocardial infarction by about 20%. Aggressive lipid lowering with statins reduces recurrent myocardial infarction by at least 30%. Thus treating hypertension in coronary patients is not the whole answer, but it is some of the answer and should therefore be treated assiduously since there are further benefits with reversal of left ventricular hypertrophy, congestive cardiac failure and a reduction in sudden cardiac death.

Principals of treatment of hypertension in patients with angina

Angina is the pain of myocardial ischemia, brought on by cardiac work which exceeds the ability of the available myocardium. Myocardial work can be measured roughly as the product of heart rate and blood pressure. It therefore follows that anti-hypertensive therapy should try and reduce both these factors.

ß-blockers are the best drugs for angina. They are in my view, unquestionably first line agents for such patients. If individuals cannot tolerate ß-blockers because of airways disease, then diltiazem or verapamil can be used, the two calcium channel blockers which reduce heart rate. Of course, fewer than half of hypertensive patients have their blood pressure treated successfully with atenolol. Once they are adequately beta blocked, i.e., their resting heart rate is about 55-65 bpm, dihydropyridine calcium channel blockers (avoiding verapamil and diltiazem) can be added.

Dihydropyridines, like nifedipine and amlodipine have a synergistic effect on reducing the effects of angina. If a third agent is required then ACE inhibitors are valuable. Although they have no effect on symptoms of angina, they improve the long term survival of such patients. Long acting nitrates and nicorandil have modest effects on blood pressure. Recently, patients with LVH have been shown to do particularly well with losartan-based therapy.

For patients with angina who are intolerant of ß-blockers a suggested regimen is to commence therapy with diltiazem, adding longacting nitrates and/or nicorandil. If blood pressure remains elevated ACE inhibitors can be added with thiazides as an addition if required. Verapamil has more sided effects, principally constipation, than diltiazem, if doses necessary to achieve good heart rate reductions are prescribed.

Hypertension and Valvular Heart Disease
Valvular heart disease usually presents now in the developed world among the elderly or middle-aged population. In developing countries rheumatic heart disease is common in early adulthood. Hypertension does not frequently accompany the typical mitral stenosis seen in developing nations. In contrast, there is an increasing population of elderly individuals who present with degenerative cardiac valve disease and often have hypertension as well.

Aortic Stenosis
We see increasingly patients who are elderly and well with a combination of aortic stenosis and hypertension. They often have a rather narrower pulse pressure than other elderly patients with systolic hypertension. Anti-hypertensive therapy must be used with caution because the heart in a stenotic patient develops tremendous pressure to squeeze the blood through the narrowed aortic orifice. Therefore the intramyocardial pressure can be very high, exceeding 200 mmHg. This affects coronary blood flow. Injudicious vasodilatation of the peripheral circulation can lead to a precipitous fall in coronary blood flow and consequent heart failure. Moreover, drugs reducing contractility should be avoided.

Therefore, for patients with aortic stenosis and hypertension ß-blockers should be avoided. Similarly, large doses of calcium channel blockers, ACE inhibitors or any other vasodilator should be avoided as initial therapy. Thiazide diuretics are the safest drugs, and tiny does of ACE inhibitors can be added if required. Titration should be very gradual. Statins may reduce the progression of aortic stenosis and are under trial.

Aortic Regurgitation
Patients with hypertension and aortic regurgitation are much easier to manage. It is likely, although not absolutely proven, that aggressive blood pressure lowering may slightly reduce the rate of progression of aortic regurgitant valve disease. The available evidence support ACE inhibitors and calcium channel blockers. Thiazide diuretics would be a useful third line.

Mitral Stenosis
Co-existing severe mitral stenosis and hypertension is unusual, since the cardiac output is low. Left ventricular function is preserved in mitral stenosis. Diuretics are often first line therapy since fluid retention is a feature of mitral valve disease. Pulmonary hypertension will develop in time in untreated patients and therapy for this with currently available drugs is not very effective. There is some hope that endothelin antagonists and selective phosphodiaesterase inhibitors might be of value.

Mitral Regurgitation
The asymptomatic patients with progressive mitral regurgitation is one of the most difficult long-term management problems in Cardiology. Such patients may seem in reasonable health for many years and then present with progressive heart failure. Crucial management involves echocardiographic follow-up; left ventricular dimensions are perhaps the most sensitive and convenient measure of progression of mitral valve disease.

Treating high blood pressure likely reduces the progression of mitral regurgitation by off-loading the left ventricle. ACE inhibitors and diuretics are first line therapy and other drugs can be added as required. LV function may look better on echocardiography than it actually is. ß-blockers should be used cautiously in severe mitral regurgitation.

Atheromatous Aortic Disease
Ruptured or bleeding abdominal aortic aneurysm is a not infrequent surgical emergency. Aortic atherosclerosis is nearly always present. Hypertension may be present beforehand. If such individuals survive major surgery, aggressive blood pressure lowering is employed together with cholesterol lowering with statins. Abdominal aortic aneurysms are usually below the renal artery although renal artery stenosis from other atheroma not infrequently co-exists. Aneuryms of the upper abdominal aorta are much less common, and thoracic aneurysm even less common.

Individuals with genetically abnormal collagen, for example Marfan's disease, develop aortic aneurysm much earlier. Beta blockade can reduce the progression of aortic dilatation and aggressive blood pressure lowering using ß-blockers with other therapy is employed. Takayasu's disease, with arteritis of major arteries frequently has co-existing hypertension from renal artery involvement. Renal artery angioplasty and anti-hypertensive therapy are indicated.

Aortic Dissection

Rupture of the aortic intima with cleavage through the medial layer of the aortic wall, is a sudden and catastrophic event. It is usually associated with aortic atheroma but hypertension frequently co-exists. In patients who survive major surgery, and patients who have a dissection extending distally from the descending thoracic aorta (who are managed conservatively without surgery), aggressive blood pressure is indicated. ß-blockers with whatever drugs are required to obtain a systolic blood pressure of between 100 – 120 mm Hg systolic are used in the acute phase of ascending aortic rupture. Emergency blood pressure lowering using intravenous sodium nitroprusside, intravenous Labetalol or the ultra-short acting esmolol can be used while plans for surgery are being made.

References

1. Braunwald E, Zypes, Libby, Heart Disease, 6th Edition, WB Saunders Company 2001

    For further reading, there are many excellent chapters in this definitive text book of Cardiology.

CHAPTER 16

24-HOUR AMBULATORY BLOOD PRESSURE MONITORING *Henry Elliott*

The recent guidelines from national and international authorities are consistent in their recommendations for "tighter" blood pressure (BP) control, particularly in patients at high risk of cardiovascular disease. "Tight" BP control applies specifically to the conventional clinical BP measurement but, increasingly, it is being recognized that consistent BP control throughout 24 hours is also a desirable target. However, rather than recommending the widespread use of repeat ambulatory blood pressure measurements (ABPM) for every hypertensive patient, the following are the principal considerations for the use of 24-hour ABPM (figure 1).

- Guidelines for the use of 24-hour ABP monitoring
- 24-hour BP values and cardiovascular morbidity and mortality
- 24-hour BP control: practical examples

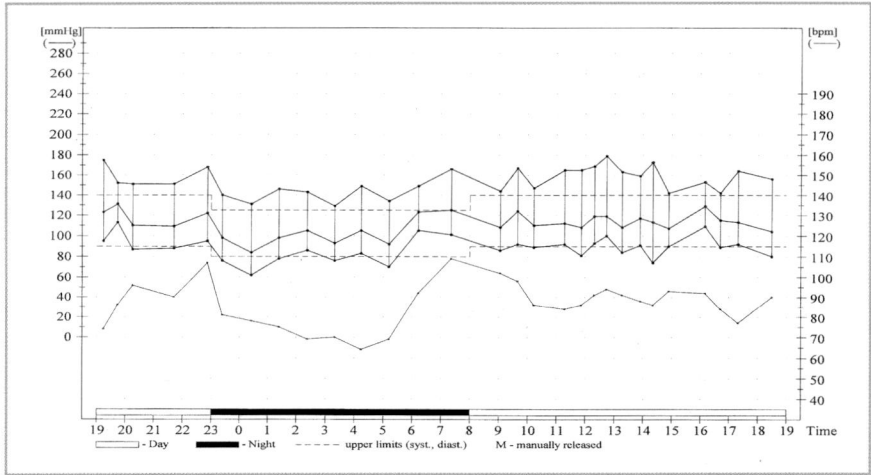

Figure 1. 24-hour ambulatory blood pressure recording of a 54-year-old woman. Note the nocturnal dip, and rise in BP before waking.

24-Hour ambulatory BP monitoring

Both the WHO/ISH and the BHS have issued guidelines concerning the current recommendations for the use of ABPM in routine clinical practice [1, 2]. While there are some differences in points of detail, the principal practical messages are consistent.

1. Prospective (outcome) data for ABPM itself are very limited and there are no outcome studies in which drug treatment has been directed in accordance with the ABPM values. In routine practice, therefore, the management decisions should continue to be based upon the conventional clinic BP reading.

2. ABPM is not (yet) recommended as part of the routine work up of every hypertensive patient but instead should be reserved for those in whom there are specific management issues, either to withhold drug treatment or to intensify it.

3. ABPM values are invariably lower than clinic BP readings. Relative to the clinic BP, the ABPM daytime average value (which is generally preferred to the full 24-hour average value) will typically be lower by 10-15mmHg systolic and 5-10mmHg diastolic BP. Because of this, treatment thresholds and targets must be adjusted downwards when making decisions based on ABPM data. Precise adjustment for an individual patient is complex but the average difference between daytime average pressures (determined by ABPM) and clinic BP is approximately 12/7mmHg. Recommended targets for ABPM values and conventional clinic BP values are shown in table 1.

Comment

The overwhelming conclusion is that ABPM is important and valuable but not recommended for indiscriminate or routine use in every hypertensive patient. Instead, ABPM is indicated when major management decisions might be implicated e.g. to withhold antihypertensive drug treatment in an otherwise low risk patient, or to intensify treatment in a high risk patient with sub-optimal BP control. In these circumstances, the information derived from the ABPM is likely to contribute to the decision making for the ongoing management of the patient.

24-Hour BP And cardiovascular morbidity and mortality

The long term consequences of uncontrolled hypertension manifest through the development of cardiovascular target organ damage. However, the predictive power of the conventional clinic BP measurement is relatively weak, whereas a number of studies have described closer relationships with the BP values derived from 24-hour ABPM. Thus, the concept has arisen that target organ damage is more likely to occur when the BP remains elevated throughout the whole 24-hour period. This concept includes the information that the persistence of an elevated overnight BP also contributes significantly to the development of target organ damage. In the research setting, 24-hour blood pressure values have been repeatedly and consistently correlated with a number of different measurements of target organ damage (table 2). Thus, it is reasonable to assume that the level of BP throughout 24 hours is the principal The importance of 24-hour BP values was first identified in the study by Perloff et al which showed that ambulatory values provided prognostic power additional to that

	Clinic BP (mmHg)		Mean daytime ABPM (mmHg)	
	No diabetes	Diabetes	No diabetes	Diabetes
Optimal BP	<140/85	<140/80	<130/80	<130/75
Audit standard	<150/90	<140/85	<140/85	<140/80

BP = blood pressure; ABPM = ambulatory blood pressure monitoring.

Source: Ramsay et al (1999)

Table 1. Treatment targets.

- Overall target organ damage score
- Left ventricular mass
- Impaired left ventricular function
- (Micro)albuminuria
- Brain damage (cerebral lacunae)
- Retinopathy
- Intima-media thickness (carotid)

Table 2. 24-h average blood pressure correlates with different types of target organ damage.

obtained by conventional BP measurements[3]. This seminal observation has since been confirmed by the results of several other studies. For example, in a study of older patients with systolic hypertension it was noted that an increment of 10mmHg in 24-hour average systolic BP average was associated with a 23% increase in total mortality and a 34% increase in cardiovascular mortality[4]. In another study in Japanese hypertensive patients, it was shown that ambulatory BP had a stronger predictive power for stroke risk than the screening (clinic) BP[5]. This latter study is arguably the only prospective study assessing the prognostic relevance of 24-hour ambulatory BP values.

Comment
There is not yet a definitive outcome trial in which treatment has been governed by the 24-hour BP values. Nevertheless, the volume of evidence is overwhelming in indicating that control of BP throughout the whole 24-hours is an appropriate goal.

24-Hour Blood Pressure Control: Practical Issues
Recent studies from the UK and USA have clearly identified the shortcomings of current antihypertensive treatment strategies insofar as less than 50% of hypertensive patients are identified and satisfactorily treated to achieve the recommended treatment targets for clinic BP. In turn, this raises the question: if clinic BP is not well controlled, how many patients have optimal control throughout 24-hours?

For example, in a study of patients with refractory hypertension the study population was sub-divided into three groups according to their average 24-hour diastolic BP[6]. These patients were all refractory to treatment with at least three antihypertensive drugs, including a thiazide diuretic, and according to the clinic values all remained uncontrolled with diastolic blood pressures above 95mmHg. However, those patients in the lowest tertile for 24-hour ABPM had an incidence of cardiovascular events at 2.2/100 patient years which was significantly lower than that seen in the middle tertile with a rate of 9.5/100 patient years and in the highest tertile with a rate of 13.6/100 years. The average 24-hour diastolic BPs were respectively less than 88mmHg, between 88 and 97mmHg and greater than 97mmHg. Thus, it was the quality of the 24-hour BP control which determined the rate of adverse events not the clinic BP which appeared similar in all patients.

Comment
This illustrates the concept that, in practice, 24 hour ABPM may help with difficult management decisions. In this example, there would be clear justification for intensifying the antihypertensive drug treatment of most of these high risk patients because they clearly demonstrated uncontrolled BP across the whole 24-hours. In contrast, the decision might deliberately (and confidently) be taken not to prescribe antihypertensive drug treatment for an otherwise low risk patient with a clinic BP of 158/98 but a daytime ABPM average BP of less than 130/80 mmHg.

Conclusions
There is no doubt that 24-hour ABPM and the derived BP values have provided additional and important insights into the relationships between hypertension and cardiovascular morbidity and mortality. Of particular practical importance is the evidence that patients at high risk can be clearly identified by 24-hour BP measurement but not always by conventional clinic BP measurement. Conversely, patients at low cardiovascular risk can also be clearly identified to the extent that reassurance is provided about a decision to withhold long term antihypertensive drug

treatment. Thus, there are the obvious practical consequences that intensified treatment can confidently be targeted to high risk patients and unnecessary treatment can be avoided in low risk patients.

The practical considerations of expense, time and resources, suggest that it is impracticable to obtain 24-hour BP measurements in every hypertensive patient and to repeat these on each occasion that a treatment change is implemented. However, to ensure that 24-hour BP control is achieved, and with the preference for once daily antihypertensive drug treatment, it follows that drugs with a protracted duration of action are to be preferred. Thus, in line with the current emphasis on "tight" BP control there is a further practical recommendation that appropriately long acting agents, either as monotherapy or in combination therapy, should be prescribed. determinant of the damage to the blood vessels of the heart, brain and kidneys.

References

1. Guidelines Committee. 1999 World Health Organisation - International Society of Hypertension Guidelines for the Management of Hypertension. J. Hypertens. 1999; 17: 151-83.

2. LE Ramsay, B Williams, GD Johnston et al. Guidelines for management of hypertension: report of the Third Working Party of the British Hypertension Society. J Hum Hypertens. 1999; 13: 569-92.

3. Perloff D, Sokolow M, Cowan R. The prognostic value of ambulatory blood pressures. JAMA. 1983; 249: 2792-8.

4. JA Staessen, L Thijs, R Fagard et al for the Systolic Hypertension in Europe Trial Investigators. Predicting cardiovascular risk using conventional vs ambulatory blood pressure in older patients with systolic hypertension. JAMA. 1999; 282: 539-46.

5. T Ohkubo, A Hozawa, K Nagai et al. Prediction of stroke by ambulatory blood pressure monitoring versus screening blood pressure measurements in a general population: the Ohasama study. J Hypertens. 2000; 18: 847-54.

6. J Redon, C Campos, ML Narciso et al. Prognostic value of ambulatory blood pressure monitoring in refractory hypertension: a prospective study. Hypertension. 1998; 31: 712-18.

CHAPTER 17

COMPLIANCE TO CONCORDANCE IN HYPERTENSION

Dean Patterson, Adrian Brady and Thomas MacDonald

Introduction

What is compliance?

Compliance is defined as a patient's behavior in terms of taking prescribed medication, following diets, or executing medically recommended lifestyle changes. Furthermore, compliance measures the extent to which a person's behavior coincides with medical advice.

Types of compliance

- Primary

  -Non-redemption of prescription[1]

- Secondary

  -Partial: self-explanatory

  -Complete: self-explanatory

  -"Toothbrush" effect: taking of tablets just prior to appointment

The incidence of non-compliance is reported as between 5% 60% [2]. Otherwise stated one third of patients always take their treatment, one third take it sometimes and one third never take their prescribed medication. It has been estimated that within the first year of treatment 16-50% of hypertensives discontinue their anti-hypertensive medications.

Is it concordance?

Concordance is an agreement reached after negotiation between a patient and a healthcare professional that respects the beliefs and wishes of the patient in determining whether, when, and how medicines are to be taken.

Concordance, however, is not a replacement for compliance. Concordance requires the agreement of two parties. If concordance is successful some patients will decide not to take their medicine and some may decide to alter their treatment, and the outcome may not be what the clinician thinks is best.

The widespread failure to control high blood pressure reflects a lack of concordance and compliance[3].

What is the most accurate way of assessing compliance?

Compliance with antihypertensive treatment is a critical factor. A standardization of the methods for recording compliance is needed especially in clinical trials. Inaccurate methods may invalidate research and clinical practice.

Research has generally failed to use valid quantitative measures of compliance. One review found only 31% of compliance studies using objective measures prior to 1978. Better measures of compliance have recently been found.

● **Direct (objective) methods**

Direct methods give a higher incidence of non-compliance than indirect methods. Blood or urine levels of the antihypertensive agent or added marker can be made or electronic pill counters used.

Assay of drug level are reliable for compliance assessment. The urinary hydrochlorothiazide-creatinine ratio (UHCR) is an accurate index of compliance for the preceding 24-hours[4]. Phenobarbitone (low dose) and riboflavin are potentially useful as pharmacological indicators of compliance with drug therapy.

At present the reference standard is electronic medication monitors. They identify various patient profiles, "omitters ", "metronome", "regular" "irregular and anarchic" patients. Their use allows the physician to adapt his management of specific problems of compliance.

● **Indirect (subjective) methods**

Indirect compliance measures include interview schedule, pill counts, blood pressure measurement and drug refill patterns.

Refill patterns are unobtrusive and easily determined, but they measure the timeliness of prescription refills, not actual drug taking. Discrepancies often exist between the medical chart, pharmacy records and verbal advice given to the patient. They should be applied cautiously over time periods of < 60 days.

Apart from electronic pill monitors patient interview has been found to be the most sensitive and accurate measure of compliance. When compared to direct assay, hydrochlorothiazide; this measure correctly classifies 85% of patients as to compliant or noncompliant.

Factors Affecting Compliance

Many problems relate to maintaining long term therapy in the hypertensive population. They include:

Patient factors-

- Male sex
- Young age
- Obesity
- Cigarette smoking
- Direct referral to the clinic as a result of screening instead of referral by a general practitioner
- Absence of pre-existing antihypertensive treatment at the first visit
- Moderate hypertension
- Low socio-economic category
- Tension, anxiety, irritability, fatigue, low mood
- Interpersonal relations problems
- Low quality of life.

Most commonly non-compliance is related to deterioration in a patient's quality of life produced by antihypertensive agents. There is increasing evidence that social and behavioral science techniques can be used to quantify this deterioration in a patient's quality of life. In one study 98% of patients wanted to know about all possible side effects of medications as well as the most likely side effects.

Pharmacological factors-

- Cost of medication,
- A lack of written instructions,
- Unclear instructions,
- Complexity of the treatment regimen
- Side effects, (urinary incontinence and in men sexual dysfunction)

The withdrawal of a significant proportion of newly diagnosed patients from therapy within the first year seems to be related to the choice of initial antihypertensive agent, with respect to drug side effects and dosing schedule. A rank order of higher to lower persistence rates after one year is ARBs, ACE inhibitors, calcium antagonists, ß-blockers and diuretics. This relation indicates the importance of real-world studies for evidence-based medicine.

Physician factors

- Non-involvement of the patient in designing the treatment plan
- Lack of patient education about the disease
- Poor doctor-patient communication
- Physician job satisfaction
- Number of patients seen per week
- Scheduling a follow-up appointment
- Number of tests ordered
- Seriousness of illness
- Patient health distress.

Four major components are involved in physician behavior that may impact on patient compliance with treatment regimens: compassion, communication, activating patient self-motivation and shared responsibility with the patient. Physician behavior is the factor most easily modified to improve compliance.[6]

What Level of Non Compliance Have Been Researched

As the incidence of non-compliance varies in hypertensive patients so it varies in different population groups. In newly diagnosed hypertensives persistence with antihypertensive therapy has been shown to be better than in older and female patients[7].

Owing to increasing rates of hypertension and cardiovascular-related diseases in developing countries, compliance with antihypertensive medication is major public health importance. Few studies have reported on compliance in developing countries. In the Seychelles, compliance improved with the level of literacy, and depended on the presence absence of diuretics in the medication. The ability of patients to report correctly the number of antihypertensive pills to be taken daily was a predictor of compliance.

In the third world setting other factors that appeared to affect patient compliance were free medication, free hospital visits, free transportation, open discussion with medical staff, use of a common dialect, and politeness of medical staff. Culturally influenced health beliefs are an important influence on compliance.

Measures To Improve Compliance

● Physician factors

Physicians should communicate instructions clearly and prescribe therapies that are effective, affordable, have minimal or no adverse effects on patient quality of life and neutral to positive effect on overall cardiac risk profile. The needs of special hypertensive populations (i.e., elderly, black, and young patients) must also be recognized and addressed. It is unlikely that any single compliance-improving strategy will adequately address the problem in all patients. Instead, combinations of techniques offered continuously over the span of the therapy are more likely to be successful. The common element that appears to run through all of the compliance studies is the attention given study patients by health workers. It may be that regardless of the specific techniques used, increasing attention to the compliance issue will help keep it in the forefront during decision-making and improve compliance behavior.

● Patient factors

Early detection of patients at high risk of drop out or poor blood pressure control might improve treatment of hypertension and allow management to be more individually adapted to each patient. Other methods of optimizing compliance include prescription-refill reminders, appointment reminders, and simple written instructions about drug use, using group exercise, nurse telephone calls, social support and patient education about the need for treatment and the consequences of non-compliance.

Occupationally based programmes that are patient-centered, supportive and provide appropriate intervention succeed 'on' or 'off' site. The lesson for conventional sources of care, wherever they exist, is to reorient the process of care and its relation to the patient to over come the disincentives to persistence in successful care.

Behavior strategies, including the tailoring of pill taking to patients' daily habits and rituals, the advocacy of self-monitoring of pills and blood pressure, and the institution of reward systems are further interventions that can improve compliance. Self-recording of blood pressure can increase compliance by 30%. We believe this to be one of the most useful means to improve compliance. Patients are given ownership of their condition and we believe self recording may be the best single measure towards better compliance.

Group therapy can be used to improve patients' knowledge of their condition, and to combat contributory factors such as obesity, smoking and high salt intake and thereby improve compliance. Patient-led organizations such as th Blood Pressure Association in the UK have an important role here.

Pharmacological factors

Numerous studies have found that compliance increases as drug-dosage frequency decreases, as with the use of once-daily or sustained-release drug preparations. Introduction of once daily treatment early in the course of antihypertensive therapy can improve compliance by the order of 30%. Correct choice of initial antihypertensive agent, with respect to drug side effects and dosing schedule will improve compliance.[8]

Other factors

Most life insurance companies are willing to reduce the cost of yearly premiums when blood pressure is successfully treated and controlled for several years. Physicians should bring these facts to their patients' attention as a motivating factor to improve adherence to therapy.

Conclusion

In determining the most appropriate antihypertensive program for an individual patient, physicians need to be able to assess the impact of the agent on quality of life in addition to the more common triad of efficacy, cost, and serious side effects. A patient's overall level of wellbeing and perception of functional capacity may be more sensitive to the pharmacologic effects of antihypertensive agents than previously recognized. Compliance may well be the ultimate determinate of success with any antihypertensive regimen. Therefore, it is essential that clinicians implement pharmacologic therapy that balances biophysiologic needs with quality-of-life considerations to achieve the most successful and viable patient outcomes. Rational medical decisions should be based on the best possible evidence. Clinical trial results, however, may not reflect conditions in actual practice. In hypertension, for example, trials indicate equivalent antihypertensive efficacy and safety for many medications, yet blood pressure frequently remains uncontrolled, perhaps owing to poor compliance.

Barriers to persistence occur early in the therapeutic course and achieving successful therapy when treatment is started is important to maintaining long term persistence.

Keypoints

1. Compliance measures the extent to which a person's behavior coincides with medical advice.

   Primary and secondary non-compliance,

   The incidence of non-compliance 5- 60%.

2. Concordance is an agreement reached after negotiation between a patient and a healthcare professional.

3. Research has generally failed to use valid quantitative measures of compliance examples of which include direct methods (Blood or urine drug levels or electronic pill counters) or indirect methods (interview schedule, pill counts, blood pressure measurement and drug refill patterns, serum ACE activity)

4. Patient, Pharmacological and Physician factors all affect compliance

5. As the incidence of non-compliance varies in hypertensive patients so it varies in different population groups.

6. Improving compliance

   Physician factors
   Communicate clearly
   Prescribe effective, affordable therapies
   No adverse effects on quality of life
   Combinations of techniques offered continuously

   Patient factors
   Early detection high-risk patients
   Occupationally based programmes
   Behavior strategies
   Self-recording of blood pressure
   Group therapy
   Prescription-refill reminders
   Appointment reminders,
   Simple written instructions about drug use
   Patient education

   Pharmacological factors
   Once-daily or sustained-release drug preparations
   Correct choice of initial antihypertensive agent,

Other factors
Life insurance premiums

7. Biophysiologic needs vs quality-of-life considerations
Barriers to persistence occur early in the therapeutic course
Achieving successful therapy when treatment is started is important to
maintaining long term persistence.

References

1. Beardon PH, McGilchrist MM, McKendrick AD, McDevitt DG, MacDonald TM. Primary non-compliance with prescribed medication in primary care [see comments]. *BMJ* 1993; 307: 846-848.

2. Jones JK, Gorkin L, Lian JF, Staffa JA, Fletcher AP. Discontinuation of and changes in treatment after start of new courses of antihypertensive drugs: a study of a United Kingdom population. *BMJ* 1995; 311: 293-295.

3. Mullen PD. Compliance becomes concordance. *BMJ* 1997; 314: 691-692.

4. Hodge RHJ, Lynch SS, Davison JP, Knight JG, Sinn JA, Carey RM. Estimating compliance with diuretic therapy: urinary hydrochlorothiazide-creatinine ratios in normal subjects. *Hypertension* 1979; 1: 537-542.

5. Struthers AD, Anderson G, MacFadyen RJ, Fraser C, MacDonald TM. Non-adherence with ACE inhibitor treatment is common in heart failure and can be detected by routine serum ACE activity assays [In Process Citation]. *Heart* 1999; 82: 584-588.

6. Coleman VR. Physician behaviour and compliance. *J Hypertens Suppl* 1985; 3: S69-S71

7. Breckenridge A. Compliance of hypertensive patients with pharmacological treatment. *Hypertension* 1983; 5: III85-III89

8. Caro JJ. Stepped care for hypertension: are the assumptions valid? *J Hypertens Suppl* 1997; 15: S35-S39

9. Fodor G, Cutler H, Irvine J, Ramsden V, Tremblay G, Chockalingam A. Adherence to non-pharmacologic therapy for hypertension: problems and solutions. Canadian Journal of Public Health 1998; Revue Canadienne de Sante Publique. 89: I12-I15

INDEX

C

I

J

K

L

R

S